SLEEP-WAKE DISORDERS

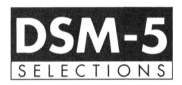

SLEEP-WAKE DISORDERS

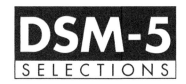

American Psychiatric Association

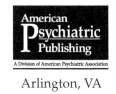

Arlington, VA

Manufactured in the United States of America on acid-free paper.

ISBN 978-1-61537-009-2 (Paperback)

American Psychiatric Association
1000 Wilson Boulevard
Arlington, VA 22209-3901
www.psych.org

Sleep-Wake Disorders: DSM-5® Selections is an anthology published by the American Psychiatric Association from the following sources:

American Psychiatric Association: *Diagnostic and Statistical Manual of Mental Disorders,* Fifth Edition. Arlington, VA, American Psychiatric Association, 2013

Black DW, Grant JE: *DSM-5® Guidebook: The Essential Companion to the Diagnostic and Statistical Manual of Mental Disorders, Fifth Edition.* Washington, DC, American Psychiatric Publishing, 2014

Barnhill JW: *DSM-5® Clinical Cases.* Washington, DC, American Psychiatric Publishing, 2014

Muskin PR: *DSM-5® Self-Exam Questions: Test Questions for the Diagnostic Criteria.* Washington, DC, American Psychiatric Publishing, 2014

Contents

Introduction to DSM-5® Selections

Welcome to *DSM-5 Selections.* The purpose of this series is to educate readers about important diagnostic issues associated with categories of DSM-5 disorders. The initial books in the *DSM-5 Selections* series are *Sleep-Wake Disorders, Depressive Disorders, Schizophrenia Spectrum and Other Psychotic Disorders, Feeding and Eating Disorders, Neurodevelopmental Disorders,* and *Anxiety Disorders.* Each book in the series includes the diagnostic criteria relevant to the disorders included in each category. The criteria are taken directly from DSM-5, the most comprehensive, current, and critical resource for clinical practice available today. Also included in each book in the series are extracts from the *DSM-5 Guidebook, DSM-5 Clinical Cases,* and *DSM-5 Self-Exam Questions.* Consequently, each book in the series offers readers a unique introduction to individual categories of DSM-5 disorders and an opportunity to test one's knowledge about DSM-5 disorders.

DSM-5 Guidebook serves as a roadmap to DSM-5 disorders for clinicians and researchers. It illuminates the content of DSM-5 by teaching mental health professionals how to use the revised diagnostic criteria, and it provides practical content for its clinical use. The book offers a fresh perspective to DSM diagnostic categories by focusing on the changes between DSM-IV-TR and DSM-5 that will most significantly impact clinical application of the criteria.

DSM-5 Clinical Cases presents composite patient cases that exemplify the diagnostic criteria for disorders contained in a category. *DSM-5 Clinical Cases* makes DSM-5 come alive for teachers, students, and clinicians. The book helps readers to understand diagnostic concepts, including symptoms, severity, comorbidities, age at onset and development, dimensionality across disorders, and gender and cultural implications.

The questions in *DSM-5 Self-Exam Questions* were written to test readers' knowledge of conceptual changes to DSM-5, specific changes to diagnoses, and the diagnostic criteria. Each question includes short answers that explain the rationale for each correct answer and contain important information on diagnostic classification, criteria sets, diagnoses, codes, severity, culture, age, and gender. The questions are helpful for preparing for various examinations.

The *DSM-5 Selections* series is not intended to replace DSM-5 or the other books from which the extracts are taken. Rather, the series is intended to give readers key selected materials that pertain directly to specific disorder categories. If you find that you require more information about a specific disorder or category of disorders, you are encouraged to examine an APP textbook or clinical manual. You can review the full list of APP titles at www.appi.org.

Robert E. Hales, M.D.
Editor-in-Chief

Preface

Sleep-wake disorders derail health and shorten longevity. They are highly prevalent, affecting an estimated 50–70 million individuals in the United States. In the general population, insomnia symptoms may be present in up to 33% of individuals, obstructive sleep apnea in about 5%, and restless leg syndrome in 5%–15%.

Sleep-wake disorders are common in patients who see a psychiatrist or primary care physician. Many sleep-wake complaints are secondary to other psychiatric or medical conditions. DSM-5 is one of three classification systems that cover sleep disorders, the other two being the *International Classification of Sleep Disorders*, Third Edition (ICSD-3), which is commonly used by sleep medicine specialists, and the *International Classification of Diseases*, which is used for billing purposes. ICSD-3 lists more than 80 sleep-wake disorders in eight general categories. DSM-5 includes eight sleep-wake disorders or disorder groups (in addition to various "other specified" or "unspecified" disorders): insomnia disorder, hypersomnolence disorder, narcolepsy, breathing-related sleep disorders (including obstructive sleep apnea hypopnea, central sleep apnea, and sleep-related hypoventilation), circadian rhythm sleep-wake disorders, parasomnias (including non–rapid eye movement [REM] sleep arousal disorder, nightmare disorder, and REM sleep behavior disorder), restless legs syndrome, and substance/medication-induced sleep disorder.

Psychiatrists have long been aware of the close association between sleep and mental health/illness. Depression is most often accompanied by disturbed sleep. Untreated insomnia can lead to depression. Disturbed sleep may foreshadow an emerging psychiatric disorder, and sleep loss may trigger a manic episode. Problems with sleep often lead to other health problems. Difficulty falling asleep, unrefreshing sleep, or snoring may predict the development of metabolic syndromes. Long-term sleep deprivation is a contributor to poor health. Patients with obstructive sleep apnea may have a higher incidence of coronary artery disease. A combination of sleep restriction and circadian disruption, as seen in shift work, may be especially problematic in terms of metabolic dysregulation.

Although widespread, sleep-wake disorders often remain unexplored if clinicians do not ask about them. Patients may describe their sleep disturbance as "I can't sleep" or "his/her snoring keeps me up." The primary symptoms of disordered sleep, such as insomnia, excessive daytime sleepiness, and disturbed sleep behavior, are usually not indicative of a specific diagnosis. For example, some people who claim to be sleepy may actually be fatigued because they are unable to sleep at night or nap during the day. Other people are night owls who do not sleep in tune with their circadian

Adapted from Reite M, Weissberg M: "Sleep-Wake Disorders," in *The American Psychiatric Publishing Textbook of Psychiatry*, 6th Edition. Edited by Hales RE, Yudofsky SC, Roberts LW. Washington, DC, American Psychiatric Publishing, 2014, pp. 607–644.

arousal symptoms. These individuals can develop insomnia and other sleep-wake disorders. The correlation between sleep-wake disorders and psychiatric illness creates a host of diagnostic pitfalls. For instance, although depression can cause sleepiness and insomnia, depression and insomnia may coexist independently and may require a separate assessment. In addition, insomnia disorder may have multiple causes and frequently patients have multiple sleep disturbances.

Because of the common nature of sleep-wake disorders and their comorbidity with other psychiatric disorders, the material presented here should prove useful for a wide range of clinicians from multiple specialties. When a patient complains of sleep disturbance, never assume that it is secondary to another psychiatric disorder; it may be a primary condition that warrants further evaluation and assessment.

Highlights of Changes From DSM-IV-TR to DSM-5

Because of the DSM-5 mandate for concurrent specification of coexisting conditions (medical and mental), sleep disorders related to another mental disorder and sleep disorder due to a general medical condition have been removed from DSM-5, and greater specification of coexisting conditions is provided for each sleep-wake disorder. This change underscores that the individual has a sleep-wake disorder warranting independent clinical attention, in addition to any medical and mental disorders that are also present, and acknowledges the bidirectional and interactive effects between sleep disorders and coexisting medical and mental disorders. This reconceptualization reflects a paradigm shift that is widely accepted in the field of sleep disorders medicine. It moves away from making causal attributions between coexisting disorders. Any additional relevant information from the prior diagnostic categories of sleep disorders related to another mental disorder and sleep disorder due to another medical condition has been integrated into the other sleep-wake disorders where appropriate.

Consequently, in DSM-5, the diagnosis of primary insomnia has been renamed insomnia disorder to avoid the differentiation of primary and secondary insomnia. DSM-5 also distinguishes narcolepsy, which is now known to be associated with hypocretin deficiency, from other forms of hypersomnolence. These changes are warranted by neurobiological and genetic evidence validating this reorganization. Finally, throughout the DSM-5 classification of sleep-wake disorders, pediatric and developmental criteria and text are integrated where existing science and considerations of clinical utility support such integration. This developmental perspective encompasses age-dependent variations in clinical presentation.

Breathing-Related Sleep Disorders

In DSM-5, breathing-related sleep disorders are divided into three relatively distinct disorders: obstructive sleep apnea hypopnea, central sleep apnea, and sleep-related hypoventilation. This change reflects the growing understanding of pathophysiology in the genesis of these disorders and, furthermore, has relevance to treatment planning.

Circadian Rhythm Sleep-Wake Disorders

The subtypes of circadian rhythm sleep-wake disorders have been expanded to include advanced sleep phase type, irregular sleep-wake type, and non-24-hour sleep-wake type, whereas the jet lag type has been removed.

Rapid Eye Movement Sleep Behavior Disorder and Restless Legs Syndrome

The use of DSM-IV "not otherwise specified" diagnoses has been reduced by designating rapid eye movement sleep behavior disorder and restless legs syndrome as independent disorders. In DSM-IV, both were included under "dyssomnia not otherwise specified." Their full diagnostic status is supported by research evidence.

DSM-5® Sleep-Wake Disorders: ICD-9-CM and ICD-10-CM Codes

Disorder	ICD-9-CM	ICD-10-CM
Insomnia Disorder	307.42	F51.01
Hypersomnolence Disorder	307.44	F51.11
Narcolepsy		
Narcolepsy without cataplexy but with hypocretin deficiency	347.00	G47.419
Narcolepsy with cataplexy but without hypocretin deficiency	347.01	G47.411
Autosomal dominant cerebellar ataxia, deafness, and narcolepsy	347.00	G47.419
Autosomal dominant narcolepsy, obesity, and type 2 diabetes	347.00	G47.419
Narcolepsy secondary to another medical condition	347.10	G47.429
Breathing-Related Sleep Disorders		
Obstructive Sleep Apnea Hypopnea	327.23	G47.33
Central Sleep Apnea		
Idiopathic central sleep apnea	327.21	G47.31
Cheyne-Stokes breathing	786.04	R06.3
Central sleep apnea comorbid with opioid use	780.57	G47.37
Sleep-Related Hypoventilation		
Idiopathic hypoventilation	327.24	G47.34
Congenital central alveolar hypoventilation	327.25	G47.35
Comorbid sleep-related hypoventilation	327.26	G47.36
Circadian Rhythm Sleep-Wake Disorders		
Delayed sleep phase type	307.45	G47.21
Advanced sleep phase type	307.45	G47.22
Irregular sleep-wake type	307.45	G47.23
Non-24-hour sleep-wake type	307.45	G47.24
Shift work type	307.45	G47.26
Unspecified type	307.45	G47.20

Disorder	ICD-9-CM	ICD-10-CM
Parasomnias		
Non–Rapid Eye Movement Sleep Arousal Disorders		
Sleepwalking type	307.46	F51.3
Sleep terror type	307.46	F51.4
Nightmare Disorder	307.47	F51.5
Rapid Eye Movement Sleep Behavior Disorder	327.42	G47.52
Restless Legs Syndrome	333.94	G25.81
Substance/Medication-Induced Sleep Disorder	See table below	
Other Specified Insomnia Disorder	780.52	G47.09
Unspecified Insomnia Disorder	780.52	G47.00
Other Specified Hypersomnolence Disorder	780.54	G47.19
Unspecified Hypersomnolence Disorder	780.54	G47.10
Other Specified Sleep-Wake Disorder	780.59	G47.8
Unspecified Sleep-Wake Disorder	780.59	G47.9

Substance/Medication-Induced Sleep Disorder

		ICD-10-CM		
	ICD-9-CM	With use disorder, mild	With use disorder, moderate or severe	Without use disorder
Alcohol	291.82	F10.182	F10.282	F10.982
Caffeine	292.85	F15.182	F15.282	F15.982
Cannabis	292.85	F12.188	F12.288	F12.988
Opioid	292.85	F11.182	F11.282	F11.982
Sedative, hypnotic, or anxiolytic	292.85	F13.182	F13.282	F13.982
Amphetamine (or other stimulant)	292.85	F15.182	F15.282	F15.982
Cocaine	292.85	F14.182	F14.282	F14.982
Tobacco	292.85	NA	F17.208	NA
Other (or unknown) substance	292.85	F19.182	F19.282	F19.982

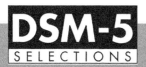

Sleep-Wake Disorders
Diagnostic and Statistical Manual of Mental Disorders, Fifth Edition

The DSM-5 classification of sleep-wake disorders is intended for use by general mental health and medical clinicians (those caring for adult, geriatric, and pediatric patients). Sleep-wake disorders encompass 10 disorders or disorder groups: insomnia disorder, hypersomnolence disorder, narcolepsy, breathing-related sleep disorders, circadian rhythm sleep-wake disorders, non–rapid eye movement (NREM) sleep arousal disorders, nightmare disorder, rapid eye movement (REM) sleep behavior disorder, restless legs syndrome, and substance/medication-induced sleep disorder. Individuals with these disorders typically present with sleep-wake complaints of dissatisfaction regarding the quality, timing, and amount of sleep. Resulting daytime distress and impairment are core features shared by all of these sleep-wake disorders.

The organization of this chapter is designed to facilitate differential diagnosis of sleep-wake complaints and to clarify when referral to a sleep specialist is appropriate for further assessment and treatment planning. The DSM-5 sleep disorders nosology uses a simple, clinically useful approach, while also reflecting scientific advances in epidemiology, genetics, pathophysiology, assessment, and interventions research since DSM-IV. In some cases (e.g., insomnia disorder), a "lumping" approach has been adopted, whereas in others (e.g., narcolepsy), a "splitting" approach has been taken, reflecting the availability of validators derived from epidemiological, neurobiological, and interventions research.

Sleep disorders are often accompanied by depression, anxiety, and cognitive changes that must be addressed in treatment planning and management. Furthermore, persistent sleep disturbances (both insomnia and excessive sleepiness) are established risk factors for the subsequent development of mental illnesses and substance use disorders. They may also represent a prodromal expression of an episode of mental illness, allowing the possibility of early intervention to preempt or to attenuate a full-blown episode.

The differential diagnosis of sleep-wake complaints necessitates a multidimensional approach, with consideration of possibly coexisting medical and neurological conditions. Coexisting clinical conditions are the rule, not the exception. Sleep disturbances furnish a clinically useful indicator of medical and neurological conditions that often coexist with depression and other common mental disorders. Prominent among these comorbidities are breathing-related sleep disorders, disorders of the heart and lungs (e.g., congestive heart failure, chronic obstructive pulmonary disease), neurodegenerative disorders (e.g., Alzheimer's disease), and disorders of the musculoskeletal system (e.g., osteoarthritis). These disorders not only may disturb sleep but also may themselves be worsened during sleep (e.g., prolonged apneas or electrocardiographic arrhythmias during REM sleep; confusional arousals in patients with dementing illness; seizures in persons with complex partial seizures). REM sleep behavior disorder is often an early indicator of neurodegenerative disorders (alpha synucleinopathies) like Parkinson's disease. For all of these reasons—related to differential diagnosis, clinical comorbidity, and facilitation of treatment planning—sleep disorders are included in DSM-5.

The approach taken to the classification of sleep-wake disorders in DSM-5 can be understood within the context of "lumping versus splitting." DSM-IV represented an effort to simplify sleep-wake disorders classification and thus aggregated diagnoses under broader, less differentiated labels. At the other pole, the *International Classification of Sleep Disorders,* 2nd Edition (ICSD-2), elaborated numerous diagnostic subtypes. DSM-IV was prepared for use by mental health and general medical clinicians who are not experts in sleep medicine. ICSD-2 reflected the science and opinions of the sleep specialist community and was prepared for use by specialists.

The weight of available evidence supports the superior performance characteristics (interrater reliability, as well as convergent, discriminant, and face validity) of simpler, less-differentiated approaches to diagnosis of sleep-wake disorders. The text accompanying each set of diagnostic criteria provides linkages to the corresponding disorders included in ICSD-2. The DSM-5 sleep-wake disorders classification also specifies corresponding nonpsychiatric listings (e.g., neurology codes) from the *International Classification of Diseases* (ICD).

The field of sleep disorders medicine has progressed in this direction since the publication of DSM-IV. The use of biological validators is now embodied in the DSM-5 classification of sleep-wake disorders, particularly for disorders of excessive sleepiness, such as narcolepsy; for breathing-related sleep disorders, for which formal sleep studies (i.e., polysomnography) are indicated; and for restless legs syndrome, which can often coexist with periodic limb movements during sleep, detectable via polysomnography.

Insomnia Disorder

Diagnostic Criteria   **307.42** (F51.01)

A. A predominant complaint of dissatisfaction with sleep quantity or quality, associated with one (or more) of the following symptoms:

   1. Difficulty initiating sleep. (In children, this may manifest as difficulty initiating sleep without caregiver intervention.)
   2. Difficulty maintaining sleep, characterized by frequent awakenings or problems returning to sleep after awakenings. (In children, this may manifest as difficulty returning to sleep without caregiver intervention.)
   3. Early-morning awakening with inability to return to sleep.

B. The sleep disturbance causes clinically significant distress or impairment in social, occupational, educational, academic, behavioral, or other important areas of functioning.

C. The sleep difficulty occurs at least 3 nights per week.

D. The sleep difficulty is present for at least 3 months.

E. The sleep difficulty occurs despite adequate opportunity for sleep.

F. The insomnia is not better explained by and does not occur exclusively during the course of another sleep-wake disorder (e.g., narcolepsy, a breathing-related sleep disorder, a circadian rhythm sleep-wake disorder, a parasomnia).

G. The insomnia is not attributable to the physiological effects of a substance (e.g., a drug of abuse, a medication).

H. Coexisting mental disorders and medical conditions do not adequately explain the predominant complaint of insomnia.

Specify if:

With non–sleep disorder mental comorbidity, including substance use disorders

With other medical comorbidity

With other sleep disorder

Coding note: The code 307.42 (F51.01) applies to all three specifiers. Code also the relevant associated mental disorder, medical condition, or other sleep disorder immediately after the code for insomnia disorder in order to indicate the association.

Specify if:

Episodic: Symptoms last at least 1 month but less than 3 months.

Persistent: Symptoms last 3 months or longer.

Recurrent: Two (or more) episodes within the space of 1 year.

Note: Acute and short-term insomnia (i.e., symptoms lasting less than 3 months but otherwise meeting all criteria with regard to frequency, intensity, distress, and/or impairment) should be coded as an other specified insomnia disorder.

Note. The diagnosis of insomnia disorder is given whether it occurs as an independent condition or is comorbid with another mental disorder (e.g., major depressive disorder), medical condition (e.g., pain), or another sleep disorder (e.g., a breathing-related sleep disorder). For instance, insomnia may develop its own course with some anxiety and depressive features but in the absence of criteria being met for any one mental disorder. Insomnia may also manifest as a clinical feature of a more predominant mental disorder. Persistent insomnia may even be a risk factor for depression and is a common residual symptom after treatment for this condition. With comorbid insomnia and a mental disorder, treatment may also need to target both conditions. Given these different courses, it is often impossible to establish the precise nature of the relationship between these clinical entities, and this relationship may change over time. Therefore, in the presence of insomnia and a comorbid disorder, it is not necessary to make a causal attribution between the two conditions. Rather, the diagnosis of insomnia disorder is made with concurrent specification of the clinically comorbid conditions. A concurrent insomnia diagnosis should only be considered when the insomnia is sufficiently severe to warrant independent clinical attention; otherwise, no separate diagnosis is necessary.

Diagnostic Features

The essential feature of insomnia disorder is dissatisfaction with sleep quantity or quality with complaints of difficulty initiating or maintaining sleep. The sleep complaints are accompanied by clinically significant distress or impairment in social, occupational, or other important areas of functioning. The sleep disturbance may occur during the course of another mental disorder or medical condition, or it may occur independently.

Different manifestations of insomnia can occur at different times of the sleep period. *Sleep-onset insomnia* (or *initial insomnia*) involves difficulty initiating sleep at bedtime. *Sleep maintenance insomnia* (or *middle insomnia*) involves frequent or prolonged awakenings throughout the night. *Late insomnia* involves early-morning awakening with an inability to return to sleep. Difficulty maintaining sleep is the most common single symptom of insomnia, followed by difficulty falling asleep, while a combination of these symptoms is the most common presentation overall. The specific type of sleep complaint often varies over time. Individuals who complain of difficulty falling asleep at one time may later complain of difficulty maintaining sleep, and vice versa. Symptoms of difficulty falling asleep and difficulty maintaining sleep can be quantified by the individual's retrospective self-report, sleep diaries, or other methods, such as actigraphy or polysomnography, but the diagnosis of insomnia disorder is based on the individual's subjective perception of sleep or a caretaker's report.

Nonrestorative sleep, a complaint of poor sleep quality that does not leave the individual rested upon awakening despite adequate duration, is a common sleep complaint usually occurring in association with difficulty initiating or maintaining sleep, or less frequently in isolation. This complaint can also be reported in association with other sleep disorders (e.g., breathing-related sleep disorder). When a complaint of nonrestorative sleep occurs in isolation (i.e., in the absence of difficulty initiating and/or maintaining sleep) but all diagnostic criteria with regard to frequency, duration, and daytime distress and impairments are otherwise met, a diagnosis of other specified insomnia disorder or unspecified insomnia disorder is made.

Aside from the frequency and duration criteria required to make the diagnosis, additional criteria are useful to quantify insomnia severity. These quantitative criteria, while arbitrary, are provided for illustrative purpose only. For instance, difficulty initiating sleep is defined by a subjective sleep latency greater than 20–30 minutes, and difficulty maintaining sleep is defined by a subjective time awake after sleep onset greater than 20–30 minutes. Although there is no standard definition of early-morning awakening, this symptom involves awakening at least 30 minutes before the scheduled time and before total sleep time reaches 6½ hours. It is essential to take into account not only the final awakening time but also the bedtime on the previous evening. Awakening at 4:00 A.M. does not have the same clinical significance in those who go to bed at 9:00 P.M. as in those who go to bed at 11:00 P.M. Such a symptom may also reflect an age-dependent decrease in the ability to sustain sleep or an age-dependent shift in the timing of the main sleep period.

Insomnia disorder involves daytime impairments as well as nighttime sleep difficulties. These include fatigue or, less commonly, daytime sleepiness; the latter is more common among older individuals and when insomnia is comorbid with another medical condition (e.g., chronic pain) or sleep disorder (e.g., sleep apnea). Impairment in cognitive performance may include difficulties with attention, concentration and memory, and even with performing simple manual skills. Associated mood disturbances are typically described as irritability or mood lability and less commonly as depressive or anxiety symptoms. Not all individuals with nighttime sleep disturbances are distressed or have functional impairment. For example, sleep continuity is often interrupted in healthy older adults who nevertheless identify themselves as good sleepers. A diagnosis of insomnia disorder should be reserved for those individuals with significant daytime distress or impairment related to their nighttime sleep difficulties.

Associated Features Supporting Diagnosis

Insomnia is often associated with physiological and cognitive arousal and conditioning factors that interfere with sleep. A preoccupation with sleep and distress due to the inability to sleep may lead to a vicious cycle: the more the individual strives to sleep, the more frustration builds and further impairs sleep. Thus, excessive attention and efforts to sleep, which override normal sleep-onset mechanisms, may contribute to the development of insomnia. Individuals with persistent insomnia may also acquire maladaptive sleep habits (e.g., spending excessive time in bed; following an erratic sleep schedule; napping) and cognitions (e.g., fear of sleeplessness; apprehensions of daytime impairments; clock monitoring) during the course of the disorder. Engaging in such activities in an environment in which the individual has frequently spent sleepless nights may further compound the conditioned arousal and perpetuate sleep difficulties. Conversely, the individual may fall asleep more easily when not trying to do so. Some individuals also report better sleep when away from their own bedrooms and their usual routines.

Insomnia may be accompanied by a variety of daytime complaints and symptoms, including fatigue, decreased energy, and mood disturbances. Symptoms of anxiety or depression that do not meet criteria for a specific mental disorder may be present, as well as an excessive focus on the perceived effects of sleep loss on daytime functioning.

Individuals with insomnia may have elevated scores on self-report psychological or personality inventories with profiles indicating mild depression and anxiety, a worrisome cognitive style, an emotion-focused and internalizing style of conflict resolution, and a somatic focus. Patterns of neurocognitive impairment among individuals with insomnia disorder are inconsistent, although there may be impairments in performing tasks of higher complexity and those requiring frequent changes in performance strategy. Individuals with insomnia often require more effort to maintain cognitive performance.

Prevalence

Population-based estimates indicate that about one-third of adults report insomnia symptoms, 10%–15% experience associated daytime impairments, and 6%–10% have symptoms that meet criteria for insomnia disorder. Insomnia disorder is the most prevalent of all sleep disorders. In primary care settings, approximately 10%–20% of individuals complain of significant insomnia symptoms. Insomnia is a more prevalent complaint among females than among males, with a gender ratio of about 1.44:1. Although insomnia can be a symptom or an independent disorder, it is most frequently observed as a comorbid condition with another medical condition or mental disorder. For instance, 40%–50% of individuals with insomnia also present with a comorbid mental disorder.

Development and Course

The onset of insomnia symptoms can occur at any time during life, but the first episode is more common in young adulthood. Less frequently, insomnia begins in childhood or adolescence. In women, new-onset insomnia may occur during menopause and persist even after other symptoms (e.g., hot flashes) have resolved. Insomnia may have a late-life onset, which is often associated with the onset of other health-related conditions.

Insomnia can be situational, persistent, or recurrent. Situational or acute insomnia usually lasts a few days or a few weeks and is often associated with life events or rapid changes in sleep schedules or environment. It usually resolves once the initial precipitating event subsides. For some individuals, perhaps those more vulnerable to sleep disturbances, insomnia may persist long after the initial triggering event, possibly because of conditioning factors and heightened arousal. The factors that precipitate insomnia may differ from those that perpetuate it. For example, an individual who is bedridden with a painful injury and has difficulty sleeping may then develop negative associations for sleep. Conditioned arousal may then persist and lead to persistent insomnia. A similar course may develop in the context of an acute psychological stress or a mental disorder. For instance, insomnia that occurs during an episode of major depressive disorder can become a focus of attention, with consequent negative conditioning, and persist even after resolution of the depressive episode. In some cases, insomnia may also have an insidious onset without any identifiable precipitating factor.

The course of insomnia may also be episodic, with recurrent episodes of sleep difficulties associated with the occurrence of stressful events. Chronicity rates range from 45% to 75% for follow-ups of 1–7 years. Even when the course of the insomnia has become chronic, there is night-to-night variability in sleep patterns, with an occasional restful night's sleep interspersed with several nights of poor sleep. The characteristics of insomnia may also change over time. Many individuals with insomnia have a history of "light" or easily disturbed sleep prior to onset of more persistent sleep problems.

Insomnia complaints are more prevalent among middle-age and older adults. The type of insomnia symptom changes as a function of age, with difficulties initiating sleep being more common among young adults and problems maintaining sleep occurring more frequently among middle-age and older individuals.

Difficulties initiating and maintaining sleep can also occur in children and adolescents, but there are more limited data on prevalence, risk factors, and comorbidity during these developmental phases of the lifespan. Sleep difficulties in childhood can result from conditioning factors (e.g., a child who does not learn to fall asleep or return to sleep without the presence of a parent) or from the absence of consistent sleep schedules and bedtime routines. Insomnia in adolescence is often triggered or exacerbated by irregular sleep schedules (e.g., phase delay). In both children and adolescents, psychological and medical factors can contribute to insomnia.

The increased prevalence of insomnia in older adults is partly explained by the higher incidence of physical health problems with aging. Changes in sleep patterns associated with the normal developmental process must be differentiated from those exceeding age-related changes. Although polysomnography is of limited value in the routine evaluation of insomnia, it may be more useful in the differential diagnosis among older adults because the etiologies of insomnia (e.g., sleep apnea) are more often identifiable in older individuals.

Risk and Prognostic Factors

While the risk and prognostic factors discussed in this section increase vulnerability to insomnia, sleep disturbances are more likely to occur when predisposed individuals are exposed to precipitating events, such as major life events (e.g., illness, separation) or less severe but more chronic daily stress. Most individuals resume normal sleep patterns after the initial triggering event has disappeared, but others—perhaps those more vulnerable to insomnia—continue experiencing persistent sleep difficulties. Perpetuating factors such as poor sleep habits, irregular sleep scheduling, and the fear of not sleeping feed into the insomnia problem and may contribute to a vicious cycle that may induce persistent insomnia.

Temperamental. Anxiety or worry-prone personality or cognitive styles, increased arousal predisposition, and tendency to repress emotions can increase vulnerability to insomnia.

Environmental. Noise, light, uncomfortably high or low temperature, and high altitude may also increase vulnerability to insomnia.

Genetic and physiological. Female gender and advancing age are associated with increased vulnerability to insomnia. Disrupted sleep and insomnia display a familial disposition. The prevalence of insomnia is higher among monozygotic twins relative to dizygotic twins; it is also higher in first-degree family members compared with the general population. The extent to which this link is inherited through a genetic predisposition, learned by observations of parental models, or established as a by-product of another psychopathology remains undetermined.

Course modifiers. Deleterious course modifiers include poor sleep hygiene practices (e.g., excessive caffeine use, irregular sleep schedules).

Gender-Related Diagnostic Issues

Insomnia is a more prevalent complaint among females than among males, with first onset often associated with the birth of a new child or with menopause. Despite higher prevalence among older females, polysomnographic studies suggest better preservation of sleep continuity and slow-wave sleep in older females than in older males.

Diagnostic Markers

Polysomnography usually shows impairments of sleep continuity (e.g., increased sleep latency and time awake after sleep onset and decreased sleep efficiency [percentage of time in bed asleep]) and may show increased stage 1 sleep and decreased stages 3 and 4 sleep. The severity of these sleep impairments does not always match the individual's clinical presentation or subjective complaint of poor sleep, as individuals with insomnia often underestimate sleep duration and overestimate wakefulness relative to polysomnography. Quantitative electroencephalographic analyses may indicate that individuals with insomnia have greater high-frequency electroencephalography power relative to good sleepers both around the sleep onset period and during non–rapid eye movement sleep, a feature suggestive of increased cortical arousal. Individuals with insomnia disorder may have a lower sleep propensity and typically do not show increased daytime sleepiness on objective sleep laboratory measures compared with individuals without sleep disorders.

Other laboratory measures show evidence, although not consistently, of increased arousal and a generalized activation of the hypothalamic-pituitary-adrenal axis (e.g., increased cortisol levels, heart rate variability, reactivity to stress, metabolic rate). In general, findings are consistent with the hypothesis that increased physiological and cognitive arousal plays a significant role in insomnia disorder.

Individuals with insomnia disorder may appear either fatigued or haggard or, conversely, overaroused and "wired." However, there are no consistent or characteristic abnormalities on physical examination. There may be an increased incidence of stress-related psychophysiological symptoms (e.g., tension headache, muscle tension or pain, gastrointestinal symptoms).

Functional Consequences of Insomnia Disorder

Interpersonal, social, and occupational problems may develop as a result of insomnia or excessive concern with sleep, increased daytime irritability, and poor concentration. Decreased attention and concentration are common and may be related to higher rates of accidents observed in insomnia. Persistent insomnia is also associated with long-term consequences, including increased risks of major depressive disorder, hypertension, and myocardial infarction; increased absenteeism and reduced productivity at work; reduced quality of life; and increased economic burden.

Differential Diagnosis

Normal sleep variations.   Normal sleep duration varies considerably across individuals. Some individuals who require little sleep ("short sleepers") may be concerned about their sleep duration. Short sleepers differ from individuals with insomnia disorder by the lack of difficulty falling or staying asleep and by the absence of characteristic daytime symptoms (e.g., fatigue, concentration problems, irritability). However, some short sleepers may desire or attempt to sleep for a longer period of time and, by prolonging time in bed, may create an insomnia-like sleep pattern. Clinical insomnia also should be distinguished from normal, age-related sleep changes. Insomnia must also be distinguished from sleep deprivation due to inadequate opportunity or circumstance for sleep resulting, for example, from an emergency or from professional or family obligations forcing the individual to stay awake.

Situational/acute insomnia.   *Situational/acute insomnia* is a condition lasting a few days to a few weeks, often associated with life events or with changes in sleep schedules. These acute or short-term insomnia symptoms may also produce significant distress and interfere with social, personal, and occupational functioning. When such symptoms are frequent enough and meet all other criteria except for the 3-month duration, a diagnosis of other specified insomnia disorder or unspecified insomnia disorder is made.

Delayed sleep phase and shift work types of circadian rhythm sleep-wake disorder. Individuals with the delayed sleep phase type of circadian rhythm sleep-wake disorder report sleep-onset insomnia only when they try to sleep at socially normal times, but they do not report difficulty falling asleep or staying asleep when their bed and rising times are delayed and coincide with their endogenous circadian rhythm. Shift work type differs from insomnia disorder by the history of recent shift work.

Restless legs syndrome. Restless legs syndrome often produces difficulties initiating and maintaining sleep. However, an urge to move the legs and any accompanying unpleasant leg sensations are features that differentiate this disorder from insomnia disorder.

Breathing-related sleep disorders. Most individuals with a breathing-related sleep disorder have a history of loud snoring, breathing pauses during sleep, and excessive daytime sleepiness. Nonetheless, as many as 50% of individuals with sleep apnea may also report insomnia symptoms, a feature that is more common among females and older adults.

Narcolepsy. Narcolepsy may cause insomnia complaints but is distinguished from insomnia disorder by the predominance of symptoms of excessive daytime sleepiness, cataplexy, sleep paralysis, and sleep-related hallucinations.

Parasomnias. Parasomnias are characterized by a complaint of unusual behavior or events during sleep that may lead to intermittent awakenings and difficulty resuming sleep. However, it is these behavioral events, rather than the insomnia per se, that dominate the clinical picture.

Substance/medication-induced sleep disorder, insomnia type. Substance/medication-induced sleep disorder, insomnia type, is distinguished from insomnia disorder by the fact that a substance (i.e., a drug of abuse, a medication, or exposure to a toxin) is judged to be etiologically related to the insomnia (see "Substance/Medication-Induced Sleep Disorder" later in this chapter). For example, insomnia occurring only in the context of heavy coffee consumption would be diagnosed as caffeine-induced sleep disorder, insomnia type, with onset during intoxication.

Comorbidity

Insomnia is a common comorbidity of many medical conditions, including diabetes, coronary heart disease, chronic obstructive pulmonary disease, arthritis, fibromyalgia, and other chronic pain conditions. The risk relationship appears to be bidirectional: insomnia increases the risk of medical conditions, and medical problems increase the risk of insomnia. The direction of the relationship is not always clear and may change over time; for this reason, comorbid insomnia is the preferred terminology in the presence of coexisting insomnia with another medical condition (or mental disorder).

Individuals with insomnia disorder frequently have a comorbid mental disorder, particularly bipolar, depressive, and anxiety disorders. Persistent insomnia represents a risk factor or an early symptom of subsequent bipolar, depressive, anxiety, and substance use disorders. Individuals with insomnia may misuse medications or alcohol to help with nighttime sleep, anxiolytics to combat tension or anxiety, and caffeine or other stimulants to combat excessive fatigue. In addition to worsening the insomnia, this type of substance use may in some cases progress to a substance use disorder.

Relationship to International Classification of Sleep Disorders

There are several distinct insomnia phenotypes relating to the perceived source of the insomnia that are recognized by the *International Classification of Sleep Disorders*, 2nd Edition (ICSD-2). These include *psychophysiological insomnia, idiopathic insomnia, sleep-state misperception,* and *inadequate sleep hygiene.* Despite their clinical appeal and heuristic value, there is limited evidence to support these distinct phenotypes.

Hypersomnolence Disorder

Diagnostic Criteria   **307.44 (F51.11)**

A. Self-reported excessive sleepiness (hypersomnolence) despite a main sleep period lasting at least 7 hours, with at least one of the following symptoms:
   1. Recurrent periods of sleep or lapses into sleep within the same day.
   2. A prolonged main sleep episode of more than 9 hours per day that is nonrestorative (i.e., unrefreshing).
   3. Difficulty being fully awake after abrupt awakening.
B. The hypersomnolence occurs at least three times per week, for at least 3 months.
C. The hypersomnolence is accompanied by significant distress or impairment in cognitive, social, occupational, or other important areas of functioning.
D. The hypersomnolence is not better explained by and does not occur exclusively during the course of another sleep disorder (e.g., narcolepsy, breathing-related sleep disorder, circadian rhythm sleep-wake disorder, or a parasomnia).
E. The hypersomnolence is not attributable to the physiological effects of a substance (e.g., a drug of abuse, a medication).
F. Coexisting mental and medical disorders do not adequately explain the predominant complaint of hypersomnolence.

Specify if:
With mental disorder, including substance use disorders
With medical condition
With another sleep disorder

Coding note: The code 307.44 (F51.11) applies to all three specifiers. Code also the relevant associated mental disorder, medical condition, or other sleep disorder immediately after the code for hypersomnolence disorder in order to indicate the association.

Specify if:
   Acute: Duration of less than 1 month.
   Subacute: Duration of 1–3 months.
   Persistent: Duration of more than 3 months.

Specify current severity:
Specify severity based on degree of difficulty maintaining daytime alertness as manifested by the occurrence of multiple attacks of irresistible sleepiness within any given day occurring, for example, while sedentary, driving, visiting with friends, or working.
   Mild: Difficulty maintaining daytime alertness 1–2 days/week.
   Moderate: Difficulty maintaining daytime alertness 3–4 days/week.
   Severe: Difficulty maintaining daytime alertness 5–7 days/week.

Diagnostic Features

Hypersomnolence is a broad diagnostic term and includes symptoms of excessive quantity of sleep (e.g., extended nocturnal sleep or involuntary daytime sleep), deteriorated quality of wakefulness (i.e., sleep propensity during wakefulness as shown by difficulty awakening or inability to remain awake when required), and sleep inertia (i.e., a period of impaired performance and reduced vigilance following awakening from the regular sleep episode or from a nap) (Criterion A). Individuals with this disorder fall asleep quickly and have a good sleep efficiency (>90%). They may have difficulty waking up in the morning, sometimes appearing confused, combative, or ataxic. This prolonged impairment of alertness at the sleep-wake transition is often referred to as *sleep inertia* (i.e., sleep drunkenness). It can also occur upon awakening from a daytime nap. During that period, the individual appears awake, but there is a decline in motor dexterity, behavior may be very inappropriate, and memory deficits, disorientation in time and space, and feelings of grogginess may occur. This period may last some minutes to hours.

The persistent need for sleep can lead to automatic behavior (usually of a very routine, low-complexity type) that the individual carries out with little or no subsequent recall. For example, individuals may find themselves having driven several miles from where they thought they were, unaware of the "automatic" driving they did in the preceding minutes. For some individuals with hypersomnolence disorder, the major sleep episode (for most individuals, nocturnal sleep) has a duration of 9 hours or more. However, the sleep is often nonrestorative and is followed by difficulty awakening in the morning. For other individuals with hypersomnolence disorder, the major sleep episode is of normal nocturnal sleep duration (6–9 hours). In these cases, the excessive sleepiness is characterized by several unintentional daytime naps. These daytime naps tend to be relatively long (often lasting 1 hour or more), are experienced as nonrestorative (i.e., unrefreshing), and do not lead to improved alertness. Individuals with hypersomnolence have daytime naps nearly everyday regardless of the nocturnal sleep duration. Subjective sleep quality may or may not be reported as good. Individuals typically feel sleepiness developing over a period of time, rather than experiencing a sudden sleep "attack." Unintentional sleep episodes typically occur in low-stimulation and low-activity situations (e.g., while attending lectures, reading, watching television, or driving long distances), but in more severe cases they can manifest in high-attention situations such as at work, in meetings, or at social gatherings.

Associated Features Supporting Diagnosis

Nonrestorative sleep, automatic behavior, difficulties awakening in the morning, and sleep inertia, although common in hypersomnolence disorder, may also be seen in a variety of conditions, including narcolepsy. Approximately 80% of individuals with hypersomnolence report that their sleep is nonrestorative, and as many have difficulties awakening in the morning. Sleep inertia, though less common (i.e., observed in 36%–50% of individuals with hypersomnolence disorder), is highly specific to hypersomnolence. Short naps (i.e., duration of less than 30 minutes) are often unrefreshing. Individuals with hypersomnolence often appear sleepy and may even fall asleep in the clinician's waiting area.

A subset of individuals with hypersomnolence disorder have a family history of hypersomnolence and also have symptoms of autonomic nervous system dysfunction, including recurrent vascular-type headaches, reactivity of the peripheral vascular system (Raynaud's phenomenon), and fainting.

Prevalence

Approximately 5%–10% of individuals who consult in sleep disorders clinics with complaints of daytime sleepiness are diagnosed as having hypersomnolence disorder. It is estimated that about 1% of the European and U.S. general population has episodes of sleep inertia. Hypersomnolence occurs with relatively equal frequency in males and females.

Development and Course

Hypersomnolence disorder has a persistent course, with a progressive evolution in the severity of symptoms. In most extreme cases, sleep episodes can last up to 20 hours. However, the average nighttime sleep duration is around 9½ hours. While many individuals with hypersomnolence are able to reduce their sleep time during working days, weekend and holiday sleep is greatly increased (by up to 3 hours). Awakenings are very difficult and accompanied by sleep inertia episodes in nearly 40% of cases. Hypersomnolence fully manifests in most cases in late adolescence or early adulthood, with a mean age at onset of 17–24 years. Individuals with hypersomnolence disorder are diagnosed, on average, 10–15 years after the appearance of the first symptoms. Pediatric cases are rare.

Hypersomnolence has a progressive onset, with symptoms beginning between ages 15 and 25 years, with a gradual progression over weeks to months. For most individuals, the course is then persistent and stable, unless treatment is initiated. The development of other sleep disorders (e.g., breathing-related sleep disorder) may worsen the degree of sleepiness. Although hyperactivity may be one of the presenting signs of daytime sleepiness in children, voluntary napping increases with age. This normal phenomenon is distinct from hypersomnolence.

Risk and Prognostic Factors

Environmental. Hypersomnolence can be increased temporarily by psychological stress and alcohol use, but they have not been documented as environmental precipitating factors. Viral infections have been reported to have preceded or accompanied hypersomnolence in about 10% of cases. Viral infections, such as HIV pneumonia, infectious mononucleosis, and Guillain-Barré syndrome, can also evolve into hypersomnolence within months after the infection. Hypersomnolence can also appear within 6–18 months following a head trauma.

Genetic and physiological. Hypersomnolence may be familial, with an autosomal-dominant mode of inheritance.

Diagnostic Markers

Nocturnal polysomnography demonstrates a normal to prolonged sleep duration, short sleep latency, and normal to increased sleep continuity. The distribution of rapid eye movement (REM) sleep is also normal. Sleep efficiency is mostly greater than 90%. Some individuals with hypersomnolence disorder have increased amounts of slow-wave sleep. The multiple sleep latency test documents sleep tendency, typically indicated by mean sleep latency values of less than 8 minutes. In hypersomnolence disorder, the mean sleep latency is typically less than 10 minutes and frequently 8 minutes or less. Sleep-onset REM periods (SOREMPs; i.e., the occurrence of REM sleep within 20 minutes of sleep onset) may be present but occur less than two times in four to five nap opportunities.

Functional Consequences of Hypersomnolence Disorder

The low level of alertness that occurs while an individual fights the need for sleep can lead to reduced efficiency, diminished concentration, and poor memory during daytime activities. Hypersomnolence can lead to significant distress and dysfunction in work and social relationships. Prolonged nocturnal sleep and difficulty awakening can result in difficulty in meeting morning obligations, such as arriving at work on time. Unintentional daytime sleep episodes can be embarrassing and even dangerous, if, for instance, the individual is driving or operating machinery when the episode occurs.

Differential Diagnosis

Normative variation in sleep. "Normal" sleep duration varies considerably in the general population. "Long sleepers" (i.e., individuals who require a greater than average amount of sleep) do not have excessive sleepiness, sleep inertia, or automatic behavior when they obtain their required amount of nocturnal sleep. Sleep is reported to be refreshing. If social or occupational demands lead to shorter nocturnal sleep, daytime symptoms may appear. In hypersomnolence disorder, by contrast, symptoms of excessive sleepiness occur regardless of nocturnal sleep duration. An inadequate amount of nocturnal sleep, or *behaviorally induced insufficient sleep syndrome,* can produce symptoms of daytime sleepiness very similar to those of hypersomnolence. An average sleep duration of fewer than 7 hours per night strongly suggests inadequate nocturnal sleep, and an average of more than 9–10 hours of sleep per 24-hour period suggests hypersomnolence. Individuals with inadequate nocturnal sleep typically "catch up" with longer sleep durations on days when they are free from social or occupational demands or on vacations. Unlike hypersomnolence, insufficient nocturnal sleep is unlikely to persist unabated for decades. A diagnosis of hypersomnolence disorder should not be made if there is a question regarding the adequacy of nocturnal sleep duration. A diagnostic and therapeutic trial of sleep extension for 10–14 days can often clarify the diagnosis.

Poor sleep quality and fatigue.   Hypersomnolence disorder should be distinguished from excessive sleepiness related to insufficient sleep quantity or quality and fatigue (i.e., tiredness not necessarily relieved by increased sleep and unrelated to sleep quantity or quality). Excessive sleepiness and fatigue are difficult to differentiate and may overlap considerably.

Breathing-related sleep disorders.   Individuals with hypersomnolence and breathing-related sleep disorders may have similar patterns of excessive sleepiness. Breathing-related sleep disorders are suggested by a history of loud snoring, pauses in breathing during sleep, brain injury, or cardiovascular disease and by the presence of obesity, oropharyngeal anatomical abnormalities, hypertension, or heart failure on physical examination. Polysomnographic studies can confirm the presence of apneic events in breathing-related sleep disorder (and their absence in hypersomnolence disorder).

Circadian rhythm sleep-wake disorders.   Circadian rhythm sleep-wake disorders are often characterized by daytime sleepiness. A history of an abnormal sleep-wake schedule (with shifted or irregular hours) is present in individuals with a circadian rhythm sleep-wake disorder.

Parasomnias.   Parasomnias rarely produce the prolonged, undisturbed nocturnal sleep or daytime sleepiness characteristic of hypersomnolence disorder.

Other mental disorders.   Hypersomnolence disorder must be distinguished from mental disorders that include hypersomnolence as an essential or associated feature. In particular, complaints of daytime sleepiness may occur in a major depressive episode, with atypical features, and in the depressed phase of bipolar disorder. Assessment for other mental disorders is essential before a diagnosis of hypersomnolence disorder is considered. A diagnosis of hypersomnolence disorder can be made in the presence of another current or past mental disorder.

Comorbidity

Hypersomnolence can be associated with depressive disorders, bipolar disorders (during a depressive episode), and major depressive disorder, with seasonal pattern. Many individuals with hypersomnolence disorder have symptoms of depression that may meet criteria for a depressive disorder. This presentation may be related to the psychosocial consequences of persistent increased sleep need. Individuals with hypersomnolence disorder are also at risk for substance-related disorders, particularly related to self-medication with stimulants. This general lack of specificity may contribute to very heterogeneous profiles among individuals whose symptoms meet the same diagnostic criteria for hypersomnolence disorder. Neurodegenerative conditions, such as Alzheimer's disease, Parkinson's disease, and multiple system atrophy, may also be associated with hypersomnolence.

Relationship to International Classification of Sleep Disorders

The *International Classification of Sleep Disorders,* 2nd Edition (ICSD-2), differentiates nine subtypes of "hypersomnias of central origin," including recurrent hypersomnia (Kleine-Levin syndrome).

Narcolepsy

Diagnostic Criteria

A. Recurrent periods of an irrepressible need to sleep, lapsing into sleep, or napping occurring within the same day. These must have been occurring at least three times per week over the past 3 months.

B. The presence of at least one of the following:

1. Episodes of cataplexy, defined as either (a) or (b), occurring at least a few times per month:

   a. In individuals with long-standing disease, brief (seconds to minutes) episodes of sudden bilateral loss of muscle tone with maintained consciousness that are precipitated by laughter or joking.

   b. In children or in individuals within 6 months of onset, spontaneous grimaces or jaw-opening episodes with tongue thrusting or a global hypotonia, without any obvious emotional triggers.

2. Hypocretin deficiency, as measured using cerebrospinal fluid (CSF) hypocretin-1 immunoreactivity values (less than or equal to one-third of values obtained in healthy subjects tested using the same assay, or less than or equal to 110 pg/mL). Low CSF levels of hypocretin-1 must not be observed in the context of acute brain injury, inflammation, or infection.

3. Nocturnal sleep polysomnography showing rapid eye movement (REM) sleep latency less than or equal to 15 minutes, or a multiple sleep latency test showing a mean sleep latency less than or equal to 8 minutes and two or more sleep-onset REM periods.

Specify whether:

347.00 (G47.419) Narcolepsy without cataplexy but with hypocretin deficiency: Criterion B requirements of low CSF hypocretin-1 levels and positive polysomnography/multiple sleep latency test are met, but no cataplexy is present (Criterion B1 not met).

347.01 (G47.411) Narcolepsy with cataplexy but without hypocretin deficiency: In this rare subtype (less than 5% of narcolepsy cases), Criterion B requirements of cataplexy and positive polysomnography/multiple sleep latency test are met, but CSF hypocretin-1 levels are normal (Criterion B2 not met).

347.00 (G47.419) Autosomal dominant cerebellar ataxia, deafness, and narcolepsy: This subtype is caused by exon 21 DNA (cytosine-5)-methyltransferase-1 mutations and is characterized by late-onset (age 30–40 years) narcolepsy (with low or intermediate CSF hypocretin-1 levels), deafness, cerebellar ataxia, and eventually dementia.

347.00 (G47.419) Autosomal dominant narcolepsy, obesity, and type 2 diabetes: Narcolepsy, obesity, and type 2 diabetes and low CSF hypocretin-1 levels have been described in rare cases and are associated with a mutation in the myelin oligodendrocyte glycoprotein gene.

347.10 (G47.429) Narcolepsy secondary to another medical condition: This subtype is for narcolepsy that develops secondary to medical conditions that cause infectious (e.g., Whipple's disease, sarcoidosis), traumatic, or tumoral destruction of hypocretin neurons.

Coding note (for ICD-9-CM code 347.10 only): Code first the underlying medical condition (e.g., 040.2 Whipple's disease; 347.10 narcolepsy secondary to Whipple's disease).

Specify current severity:

Mild: Infrequent cataplexy (less than once per week), need for naps only once or twice per day, and less disturbed nocturnal sleep.

Moderate: Cataplexy once daily or every few days, disturbed nocturnal sleep, and need for multiple naps daily.

Severe: Drug-resistant cataplexy with multiple attacks daily, nearly constant sleepiness, and disturbed nocturnal sleep (i.e., movements, insomnia, and vivid dreaming).

Subtypes

In narcolepsy without cataplexy but with hypocretin deficiency, unclear "cataplexy-like" symptoms may be reported (e.g., the symptoms are not triggered by emotions and are unusually long lasting). In extremely rare cases, cerebrospinal fluid (CSF) levels of hypocretin-1 are low, and polysomnographic/multiple sleep latency test (MSLT) results are negative: repeating the test is advised before establishing the subtype diagnosis. In narcolepsy with cataplexy but without hypocretin deficiency, test results for human leukocyte antigen (HLA) DQB1*06:02 may be negative. Seizures, falls of other origin, and conversion disorder (functional neurological symptom disorder) should be excluded. In narcolepsy secondary to infectious (e.g., Whipple's disease, sarcoidosis), traumatic, or tumoral destruction of hypocretin neurons, test results for HLA DQB1*06:02 may be positive and may result from the insult triggering the autoimmune process. In other cases, the destruction of hypocretin neurons may be secondary to trauma or hypothalamic surgery. Head trauma or infections of the central nervous system can, however, produce transitory decreases in CSF hypocretin-1 levels without hypocretin cell loss, complicating the diagnosis.

Diagnostic Features

The essential features of sleepiness in narcolepsy are recurrent daytime naps or lapses into sleep. Sleepiness typically occurs daily but must occur at a minimum three times a week for at least 3 months (Criterion A). Narcolepsy generally produces cataplexy, which most commonly presents as brief episodes (seconds to minutes) of sudden, bilateral loss of muscle tone precipitated by emotions, typically laughing and joking. Muscles affected may include those of the neck, jaw, arms, legs, or whole body, resulting in head bobbing, jaw dropping, or complete falls. Individuals are awake and aware during cataplexy. To meet Criterion B1(a), cataplexy must be triggered by laughter or joking and must occur at least a few times per month when the condition is untreated or in the past.

Cataplexy should not be confused with "weakness" occurring in the context of athletic activities (physiological) or exclusively after unusual emotional triggers such as stress or anxiety (suggesting possible psychopathology). Episodes lasting hours or days, or those not triggered by emotions, are unlikely to be cataplexy, nor is rolling on the floor while laughing hysterically.

In children close to onset, genuine cataplexy can be atypical, affecting primarily the face, causing grimaces or jaw opening with tongue thrusting ("cataplectic faces"). Alternatively, cataplexy may present as low-grade continuous hypotonia, yielding a wobbling walk. In these cases, Criterion B1(b) can be met in children or in individuals within 6 months of a rapid onset.

Narcolepsy-cataplexy nearly always results from the loss of hypothalamic hypocretin (orexin)–producing cells, causing hypocretin deficiency (less than or equal to one-third of control values, or 110 pg/mL in most laboratories). Cell loss is likely autoimmune, and approximately 99% of affected individuals carry HLA-DQB1*06:02 (vs. 12%–38% of control subjects). Thus, checking for the presence of DQB1*06:02 prior to a lumbar puncture for evaluation of CSF hypocretin-1 immunoreactivity may be useful. Rarely, low CSF levels of hypocretin-1 occur without cataplexy, notably in youths who may develop cataplexy later. CSF hypocretin-1 measurement represents the gold standard, excepting associated severe conditions (neurological, inflammatory, infectious, trauma) that can interfere with the assay.

A nocturnal polysomnographic sleep study followed by an MSLT can also be used to confirm the diagnosis (Criterion B3). These tests must be performed after the individual has stopped all psychotropic medications, following 2 weeks of adequate sleep time (as documented with sleep diaries, actigraphy). Short rapid eye movement (REM) latency (sleep-onset REM period, REM latency less than or equal to 15 minutes) during polysomnography is sufficient to confirm the diagnosis and meets Criterion B3. Alternatively, the MSLT result must be positive, showing a mean sleep latency of less than or equal to 8 minutes and two or more sleep-onset REM periods in four to five naps.

Associated Features Supporting Diagnosis

When sleepiness is severe, automatic behaviors may occur, with the individual continuing his or her activities in a semi-automatic, hazelike fashion without memory or consciousness. Approximately 20%–60% of individuals experience vivid hypnagogic hallucinations before or upon falling asleep or hypnopompic hallucinations just after awakening. These hallucinations are distinct from the less vivid, nonhallucinatory dreamlike mentation at sleep onset that occurs in normal sleepers. Nightmares and vivid dreaming are also frequent in narcolepsy, as is REM sleep behavior disorder. Approximately 20%–60% of individuals experience sleep paralysis upon falling asleep or awakening, leaving them awake but unable to move or speak. However, many normal sleepers also report sleep paralysis, especially with stress or sleep deprivation. Nocturnal eating may occur. Obesity is common. Nocturnal sleep disruption with frequent long or short awakenings is common and can be disabling.

Individuals may appear sleepy or fall asleep in the waiting area or during clinical examination. During cataplexy, individuals may slump in a chair and have slurred speech or drooping eyelids. If the clinician has time to check reflexes during cataplexy (most attacks are less than 10 seconds), reflexes are abolished—an important finding distinguishing genuine cataplexy from conversion disorder.

Prevalence

Narcolepsy-cataplexy affects 0.02%–0.04% of the general population in most countries. Narcolepsy affects both genders, with possibly a slight male preponderance.

Development and Course

Onset is typically in children and adolescents/young adults but rarely in older adults. Two peaks of onset are suggested, at ages 15–25 years and ages 30–35 years. Onset can be abrupt or progressive (over years). Severity is highest when onset is abrupt in children, and then decreases with age or with treatment, so that symptoms such as cataplexy can occasionally disappear. Abrupt onset in young, prepubescent children can be associated with obesity and premature puberty, a phenotype more frequently observed since 2009. In adolescents, onset is more difficult to pinpoint. Onset in adults is often unclear, with some individuals reporting having had excessive sleepiness since birth. Once the disorder has manifested, the course is persistent and lifelong.

In 90% of cases, the first symptom to manifest is sleepiness or increased sleep, followed by cataplexy (within 1 year in 50% of cases, within 3 years in 85%). Sleepiness, hypnagogic hallucinations, vivid dreaming, and REM sleep behavior disorder (excessive movements during REM sleep) are early symptoms. Excessive sleep rapidly progresses to an inability to stay awake during the day, and to maintain good sleep at night, without a clear increase in total 24-hour sleep needs. In the first months, cataplexy may be atypical, especially in children. Sleep paralysis usually develops around puberty in children with prepubertal onset. Exacerbations of symptoms suggest lack of compliance with medications or development of a concurrent sleep disorder, notably sleep apnea.

Young children and adolescents with narcolepsy often develop aggression or behavioral problems secondary to sleepiness and/or nighttime sleep disruption. Workload and social pressure increase through high school and college, reducing available sleep time at night. Pregnancy does not seem to modify symptoms consistently. After retirement, individuals typically have more opportunity for napping, reducing the need for stimulants. Maintaining a regular schedule benefits individuals at all ages.

Risk and Prognostic Factors

Temperamental. Parasomnias, such as sleepwalking, bruxism, REM sleep behavior disorder, and enuresis, may be more common in individuals who develop narcolepsy. Individuals commonly report that they need more sleep than other family members.

Environmental. Group A streptococcal throat infection, influenza (notably pandemic H1N1 2009), or other winter infections are likely triggers of the autoimmune process, producing narcolepsy a few months later. Head trauma and abrupt changes in sleep-wake patterns (e.g., job changes, stress) may be additional triggers.

Genetic and physiological. Monozygotic twins are 25%–32% concordant for narcolepsy. The prevalence of narcolepsy is 1%–2% in first-degree relatives (a 10- to 40-fold increase overall). Narcolepsy is strongly associated with DQB1*06:02 (99% vs. 12%–38% in control subjects of various ethnic groups; 25% in the general U.S. population). DQB1*03:01 increases, while DQB1*05:01, DQB1*06:01, and DQB1*06:03 reduce risk in the presence of DQB1*06:02, but the effect is small. Polymorphisms within the T-cell receptor alpha gene and other immune modulating genes also modulate risk slightly.

Culture-Related Diagnostic Issues

Narcolepsy has been described in all ethnic groups and in many cultures. Among African Americans, more cases present without cataplexy or with atypical cataplexy, complicating diagnosis, especially in the presence of obesity and obstructive sleep apnea.

Diagnostic Markers

Functional imaging suggests impaired hypothalamic responses to humorous stimuli. Nocturnal polysomnography followed by an MSLT is used to confirm the diagnosis of narcolepsy, especially when the disorder is first being diagnosed and before treatment has begun, and if hypocretin deficiency has not been documented biochemically. The polysomnography/MSLT should be performed after the individual is no longer taking any psychotropic drugs and after regular sleep-wake patterns, without shift work or sleep deprivation, have been documented.

A sleep-onset REM period during the polysomnography (REM sleep latency less than or equal to 15 minutes) is highly specific (approximately 1% positive in control subjects) but moderately sensitive (approximately 50%). A positive MSLT result displays an average sleep latency of less than or equal to 8 minutes, and sleep-onset REM periods in two or more naps on a four- or five-nap test. The MSLT result is positive in 90%–95% of individuals with narcolepsy versus 2%–4% of control subjects or individuals with other sleep disorders. Additional polysomnographic findings often include frequent arousals, decreased sleep efficiency, and increased stage 1 sleep. Periodic limb movements (found in about 40% of individuals with narcolepsy) and sleep apnea are often noted.

Hypocretin deficiency is demonstrated by measuring CSF hypocretin-1 immunoreactivity. The test is particularly useful in individuals with suspected conversion disorder and those without typical cataplexy, or in treatment-refractory cases. The diagnostic value of the test is not affected by medications, sleep deprivation, or circadian time, but the findings are uninterpretable when the individual is severely ill with a concurrent infection or head trauma or is comatose. CSF cytology, protein, and glucose are within normal range even when sampled within weeks of rapid onset. CSF hypocretin-1 in these incipient cases is typically already very diminished or undetectable.

Functional Consequences of Narcolepsy

Driving and working are impaired, and individuals with narcolepsy should avoid jobs that place themselves (e.g., working with machinery) or others (e.g., bus driver, pilot) in danger. Once the narcolepsy is controlled with therapy, patients can usually drive, although rarely long distances alone. Untreated individuals are also at risk for social isolation and accidental injury to themselves or others. Social relations may suffer as these individuals strive to avert cataplexy by exerting control over emotions.

Differential Diagnosis

Other hypersomnias.   Hypersomnolence and narcolepsy are similar with respect to the degree of daytime sleepiness, age at onset, and stable course over time but can be distinguished based on distinctive clinical and laboratory features. Individuals with hypersomnolence typically have longer and less disrupted nocturnal sleep, greater difficulty awakening, more persistent daytime sleepiness (as opposed to more discrete "sleep attacks" in narcolepsy), longer and less refreshing daytime sleep episodes, and little or no dreaming during daytime naps. By contrast, individuals with narcolepsy have cataplexy and recurrent intrusions of elements of REM sleep into the transition between sleep and wakefulness (e.g., sleep-related hallucinations and sleep paralysis). The MSLT typically demonstrates shorter sleep latencies (i.e., greater physiological sleepiness) as well as the presence of multiple sleep-onset REM periods in individuals with narcolepsy.

Sleep deprivation and insufficient nocturnal sleep.   Sleep deprivation and insufficient nocturnal sleep are common in adolescents and shift workers. In adolescents, difficulties falling asleep at night are common, causing sleep deprivation. The MSLT result may be positive if conducted while the individual is sleep deprived or while his or her sleep is phase delayed.

Sleep apnea syndromes.   Sleep apneas are especially likely in the presence of obesity. Because obstructive sleep apnea is more frequent than narcolepsy, cataplexy may be overlooked (or absent), and the individual is assumed to have obstructive sleep apnea unresponsive to usual therapies.

Major depressive disorder.   Narcolepsy or hypersomnia may be associated or confused with depression. Cataplexy is not present in depression. The MSLT results are most often normal, and there is dissociation between subjective and objective sleepiness, as measured by the mean sleep latency during the MSLT.

Conversion disorder (functional neurological symptom disorder).   Atypical features, such as long-lasting cataplexy or unusual triggers, may be present in conversion disorder (functional neurological symptom disorder). Individuals may report sleeping and dreaming, yet the MSLT does not show the characteristic sleep-onset REM period. Full-blown, long-lasting pseudocataplexy may occur during consultation, allowing the examining physician enough time to verify reflexes, which remain intact.

Attention-deficit/hyperactivity disorder or other behavioral problems. In children and adolescents, sleepiness can cause behavioral problems, including aggressiveness and inattention, leading to a misdiagnosis of attention-deficit/hyperactivity disorder.

Seizures. In young children, cataplexy can be misdiagnosed as seizures. Seizures are not commonly triggered by emotions, and when they are, the trigger is not usually laughing or joking. During a seizure, individuals are more likely to hurt themselves when falling. Seizures characterized by isolated atonia are rarely seen in isolation of other seizures, and they also have signatures on the electroencephalogram.

Chorea and movement disorders. In young children, cataplexy can be misdiagnosed as chorea or pediatric autoimmune neuropsychiatric disorders associated with streptococcal infections, especially in the context of a strep throat infection and high antistreptolysin O antibody levels. Some children may have an overlapping movement disorder close to onset of the cataplexy.

Schizophrenia. In the presence of florid and vivid hypnagogic hallucinations, individuals may think these experiences are real—a feature that suggests schizophrenia. Similarly, with stimulant treatment, persecutory delusions may develop. If cataplexy is present, the clinician should first assume that these symptoms are secondary to narcolepsy before considering a co-occurring diagnosis of schizophrenia.

Comorbidity

Narcolepsy can co-occur with bipolar, depressive, and anxiety disorders, and in rare cases with schizophrenia. Narcolepsy is also associated with increased body mass index or obesity, especially when the narcolepsy is untreated. Rapid weight gain is common in young children with a sudden disease onset. Comorbid sleep apnea should be considered if there is a sudden aggravation of preexisting narcolepsy.

Relationship to International Classification of Sleep Disorders

The *International Classification of Sleep Disorders*, 2nd Edition (ICSD-2), differentiates five subtypes of narcolepsy.

Breathing-Related Sleep Disorders

The breathing-related sleep disorders category encompasses three relatively distinct disorders: obstructive sleep apnea hypopnea, central sleep apnea, and sleep-related hypoventilation.

Obstructive Sleep Apnea Hypopnea

Diagnostic Criteria   **327.23 (G47.33)**

A. Either (1) or (2):

  1. Evidence by polysomnography of at least five obstructive apneas or hypopneas per hour of sleep and either of the following sleep symptoms:

    a. Nocturnal breathing disturbances: snoring, snorting/gasping, or breathing pauses during sleep.

    b. Daytime sleepiness, fatigue, or unrefreshing sleep despite sufficient opportunities to sleep that is not better explained by another mental disorder (including a sleep disorder) and is not attributable to another medical condition.

  2. Evidence by polysomnography of 15 or more obstructive apneas and/or hypopneas per hour of sleep regardless of accompanying symptoms.

Specify current severity:

  Mild: Apnea hypopnea index is less than 15.

  Moderate: Apnea hypopnea index is 15–30.

  Severe: Apnea hypopnea index is greater than 30.

Specifiers

Disease severity is measured by a count of the number of apneas plus hypopneas per hour of sleep (apnea hypopnea index) using polysomnography or other overnight monitoring. Overall severity is also informed by levels of nocturnal desaturation and sleep fragmentation (measured by brain cortical arousal frequency and sleep stages) and degree of associated symptoms and daytime impairment. However, the exact number and thresholds may vary according to the specific measurement techniques used, and these numbers may change over time. Regardless of the apnea hypopnea index (count) per se, the disorder is considered to be more severe when apneas and hypopneas are accompanied by significant oxygen hemoglobin desaturation (e.g., when more than 10% of the sleep time is spent at desaturation levels of less than 90%) or when sleep is severely fragmented as shown by an elevated arousal index (arousal index greater than 30) or reduced stages in deep sleep (e.g., percentage stage N3 [slow-wave sleep] less than 5%).

Diagnostic Features

Obstructive sleep apnea hypopnea is the most common breathing-related sleep disorder. It is characterized by repeated episodes of upper (pharyngeal) airway obstruction (apneas and hypopneas) during sleep. *Apnea* refers to the total absence of airflow, and *hypopnea* refers to a reduction in airflow. Each apnea or hypopnea represents a reduction in breathing of at least 10 seconds in duration in adults or two missed breaths in children and is typically associated with drops in oxygen saturation of 3% or greater and/or an electroencephalographic arousal. Both sleep-related (nocturnal) and wake-time symptoms are common. The cardinal symptoms of obstructive sleep apnea hypopnea are snoring and daytime sleepiness.

Obstructive sleep apnea hypopnea in adults is diagnosed on the basis of polysomnographic findings and symptoms. The diagnosis is based on symptoms of 1) nocturnal breathing disturbances (i.e., snoring, snorting/gasping, breathing pauses during sleep), or 2) daytime sleepiness, fatigue, or unrefreshing sleep despite sufficient opportunities to sleep that are not better explained by another mental disorder and not attributable to another medical condition, along with 3) evidence by polysomnography of five or more obstructive apneas or hypopneas per hour of sleep (Criterion A1). Diagnosis can be made in the absence of these symptoms if there is evidence by polysomnography of 15 or more obstructive apneas and/or hypopneas per hour of sleep (Criterion A2).

Specific attention to disturbed sleep occurring in association with snoring or breathing pauses and physical findings that increase risk of obstructive sleep apnea hypopnea (e.g., central obesity, crowded pharyngeal airway, elevated blood pressure) is needed to reduce the chance of misdiagnosing this treatable condition.

Associated Features Supporting Diagnosis

Because of the frequency of nocturnal awakenings that occur with obstructive sleep apnea hypopnea, individuals may report symptoms of insomnia. Other common, though nonspecific, symptoms of obstructive sleep apnea hypopnea are heartburn, nocturia, morning headaches, dry mouth, erectile dysfunction, and reduced libido. Rarely, individuals may complain of difficulty breathing while lying supine or sleeping. Hypertension may occur in more than 60% of individuals with obstructive sleep apnea hypopnea.

Prevalence

Obstructive sleep apnea hypopnea is a very common disorder, affecting at least 1%–2% of children, 2%–15% of middle-age adults, and more than 20% of older individuals. In the general community, prevalence rates of undiagnosed obstructive sleep apnea hypopnea may be very high in elderly individuals. Since the disorder is strongly associated with obesity, increases in obesity rates are likely to be accompanied by an increased prevalence of this disorder. Prevalence may be particularly high among males, older adults, and certain racial/ethnic groups. In adults, the male-to-female ratio of obstructive sleep apnea hypopnea ranges from 2:1 to 4:1. Gender differences decline in older age, possibly because of an increased prevalence in females after menopause. There is no gender difference among prepubertal children.

Development and Course

The age distribution of obstructive sleep apnea hypopnea likely follows a **J**-shaped distribution. There is a peak in children ages 3–8 years when the nasopharynx may be compromised by a relatively large mass of tonsillar tissue compared with the size of the upper airway. With growth of the airway and regression of lymphoid tissue during later childhood, there is reduction in prevalence. Then, as obesity prevalence increases in midlife and females enter menopause, obstructive sleep apnea hypopnea again increases. The course in older age is unclear; the disorder may level off after age 65 years, but in other individuals, prevalence may increase with aging. Because there is some age dependency of the occurrence of apneas and hypopneas, polysomnographic results must be interpreted in light of other clinical data. In particular, significant clinical symptoms of insomnia or hypersomnia should be investigated regardless of the individual's age.

Obstructive sleep apnea hypopnea usually has an insidious onset, gradual progression, and persistent course. Typically the loud snoring has been present for many years, often since childhood, but an increase in its severity may lead the individual to seek evaluation. Weight gain may precipitate an increase in symptoms. Although obstructive sleep apnea hypopnea can occur at any age, it most commonly manifests among individuals ages 40–60 years. Over 4–5 years, the average apnea hypopnea index increases in adults and older individuals by approximately two apneas/hypopneas per hour. The apnea hypopnea index is increased and incident obstructive sleep apnea hypopnea is greater among individuals who are older, who are male, or who have a higher baseline body mass index (BMI) or increase their BMI over time. Spontaneous resolution of obstructive sleep apnea hypopnea has been reported with weight loss, particularly after bariatric surgery. In children, seasonal variation in obstructive sleep apnea hypopnea has been observed, as has improvement with overall growth.

In young children, the signs and symptoms of obstructive sleep apnea hypopnea may be more subtle than in adults, making diagnosis more difficult to establish. Polysomnography is useful in confirming diagnosis. Evidence of fragmentation of sleep on the polysomnogram may not be as apparent as in studies of older individuals, possibly because of the high homeostatic drive in young individuals. Symptoms such as snoring are usually parent-reported and thus have reduced sensitivity. Agitated arousals and unusual sleep postures, such as sleeping on the hands and knees, may occur. Nocturnal enuresis also may occur and should raise the suspicion of obstructive sleep apnea hypopnea if it recurs in a child who was previously dry at night. Children may also manifest excessive daytime sleepiness, although this is not as common or pronounced as in adults. Daytime mouth breathing, difficulty in swallowing, and poor speech articulation are also common features in children. Children younger than 5 years more often present with nighttime symptoms, such as observed apneas or labored breathing, than with behavioral symptoms (i.e., the nighttime symptoms are more noticeable and more often bring the child to clinical attention). In children older than 5 years, daytime symptoms such as sleepiness and behavioral problems (e.g., impulsivity and hyperactivity), attention-deficit/hyperactivity disorder, learning difficulties, and morning headaches are more often the focus of concern. Children with obstructive sleep apnea hypopnea also may present with failure to thrive and developmental delays. In young children, obesity is a less common risk factor, while delayed growth and "failure to thrive" may be present.

Risk and Prognostic Factors

Genetic and physiological. The major risk factors for obstructive sleep apnea hypopnea are obesity and male gender. Others include maxillary-mandibular retrognathia or micrognathia, positive family history of sleep apnea, genetic syndromes that reduce upper airway patency (e.g., Down's syndrome, Treacher Collin's syndrome), adenotonsillar hypertrophy (especially in young children), menopause (in females), and various endocrine syndromes (e.g., acromegaly). Compared with premenopausal females, males are at increased risk for obstructive sleep apnea hypopnea, possibly reflecting the influences of sex hormones on ventilatory control and body fat distribution, as well as because of gender differences in airway structure. Medications for mental disorders and medical conditions that tend to induce somnolence may worsen the course of apnea symptoms if these medications are not managed carefully.

Obstructive sleep apnea hypopnea has a strong genetic basis, as evidenced by the significant familial aggregation of the apnea hypopnea index. The prevalence of obstructive sleep apnea hypopnea is approximately twice as high among the first-degree relatives of probands with obstructive sleep apnea hypopnea as compared with members of control families. One-third of the variance in the apnea hypopnea index is explained by shared familial factors. Although genetic markers with diagnostic or prognostic value are not yet available for use, eliciting a family history of obstructive sleep apnea hypopnea should increase the clinical suspicion for the disorder.

Culture-Related Diagnostic Issues

There is a potential for sleepiness and fatigue to be reported differently across cultures. In some groups, snoring may be considered a sign of health and thus may not trigger concerns. Individuals of Asian ancestry may be at increased risk for obstructive sleep apnea hypopnea despite relatively low BMI, possibly reflecting the influence of craniofacial risk factors that narrow the nasopharynx.

Gender-Related Diagnostic Issues

Females may more commonly report fatigue rather than sleepiness and may under-report snoring.

Diagnostic Markers

Polysomnography provides quantitative data on frequency of sleep-related respiratory disturbances and associated changes in oxygen saturation and sleep continuity. Polysomnographic findings in children differ from those in adults in that children demonstrate labored breathing, partial obstructive hypoventilation with cyclical desaturations, hypercapnia and paradoxical movements. Apnea hypopnea index levels as low as 2 are used to define thresholds of abnormality in children.

Arterial blood gas measurements while the individual is awake are usually normal, but some individuals can have waking hypoxemia or hypercapnia. This pattern should alert the clinician to the possibility of coexisting lung disease or hypoventilation. Imaging procedures may reveal narrowing of the upper airway. Cardiac testing may show evidence of impaired ventricular function. Individuals with severe nocturnal oxygen desaturation may also have elevated hemoglobin or hematocrit values. Validated sleep measures (e.g., multiple sleep latency test [MSLT], maintenance of wakefulness test) may identify sleepiness.

Functional Consequences of Obstructive Sleep Apnea Hypopnea

More than 50% of individuals with moderate to severe obstructive sleep apnea hypopnea report symptoms of daytime sleepiness. A twofold increased risk of occupational accidents has been reported in association with symptoms of snoring and sleepiness. Motor vehicle crashes also have been reported to be as much as sevenfold higher among individuals with elevated apnea hypopnea index values. Clinicians should be cognizant of state government requirements for reporting this disorder, especially in relationship to commercial drivers. Reduced scores on measures of health-related quality of life are common in individuals with obstructive sleep apnea hypopnea, with the largest decrements observed in the physical and vitality subscales.

Differential Diagnosis

Primary snoring and other sleep disorders.　Individuals with obstructive sleep apnea hypopnea must be differentiated from individuals with primary snoring (i.e., otherwise asymptomatic individuals who snore and do not have abnormalities on overnight polysomnography). Individuals with obstructive sleep apnea hypopnea may additionally report nocturnal gasping and choking. The presence of sleepiness or other daytime symptoms not explained by other etiologies suggests the diagnosis of obstructive sleep apnea hypopnea, but this differentiation requires polysomnography. Definitive differential diagnosis between hypersomnia, central sleep apnea, sleep-related hypoventilation, and obstructive sleep apnea hypopnea also requires polysomnographic studies.

Obstructive sleep apnea hypopnea must be differentiated from other causes of sleepiness, such as narcolepsy, hypersomnia, and circadian rhythm sleep disorders. Obstructive sleep apnea hypopnea can be differentiated from narcolepsy by the absence of cataplexy, sleep-related hallucinations, and sleep paralysis and by the presence of loud snoring, gasping during sleep, or observed apneas in sleep. Daytime sleep episodes in narcolepsy are characteristically shorter, more refreshing, and more often associated with dreaming. Obstructive sleep apnea hypopnea shows characteristic apneas and hypopneas and oxygen desaturation during nocturnal polysomnographic studies. Narcolepsy results in multiple sleep-onset rapid eye movement (REM) periods during the MSLT. Narcolepsy, like obstructive sleep apnea hypopnea, may be associated with obesity, and some individuals have concurrent narcolepsy and obstructive sleep apnea hypopnea. A diagnosis of narcolepsy does not exclude the diagnosis of obstructive sleep apnea hypopnea, as the two conditions may co-occur.

Insomnia disorder.　For individuals complaining of difficulty initiating or maintaining sleep or early-morning awakenings, insomnia disorder can be differentiated from obstructive sleep apnea hypopnea by the absence of snoring and the absence of the history, signs, and symptoms characteristic of the latter disorder. However, insomnia and obstructive sleep apnea hypopnea may coexist, and if so, both disorders may need to be addressed concurrently to improve sleep.

Panic attacks.   Nocturnal panic attacks may include symptoms of gasping or choking during sleep that may be difficult to distinguish clinically from obstructive sleep apnea hypopnea. However, the lower frequency of episodes, intense autonomic arousal, and lack of excessive sleepiness differentiate nocturnal panic attacks from obstructive sleep apnea hypopnea. Polysomnography in individuals with nocturnal panic attacks does not reveal the typical pattern of apneas or oxygen desaturation characteristic of obstructive sleep apnea hypopnea. Individuals with obstructive sleep apnea hypopnea do not provide a history of daytime panic attacks.

Attention-deficit/hyperactivity disorder.   Attention-deficit/hyperactivity disorder in children may include symptoms of inattention, academic impairment, hyperactivity, and internalizing behaviors, all of which may also be symptoms of childhood obstructive sleep apnea hypopnea. The presence of other symptoms and signs of childhood obstructive sleep apnea hypopnea (e.g., labored breathing or snoring during sleep and adenotonsillar hypertrophy) would suggest the presence of obstructive sleep apnea hypopnea. Obstructive sleep apnea hypopnea and attention-deficit/hyperactivity disorder may commonly co-occur, and there may be causal links between them; therefore, risk factors such as enlarged tonsils, obesity, or a family history of sleep apnea may help alert the clinician to their co-occurrence.

Substance/medication-induced insomnia or hypersomnia.   Substance use and substance withdrawal (including medications) can produce insomnia or hypersomnia. A careful history is usually sufficient to identify the relevant substance/medication, and follow-up shows improvement of the sleep disturbance after discontinuation of the substance/medication. In other cases, the use of a substance/medication (e.g., alcohol, barbiturates, benzodiazepines, tobacco) has been shown to exacerbate obstructive sleep apnea hypopnea. An individual with symptoms and signs consistent with obstructive sleep apnea hypopnea should receive that diagnosis, even in the presence of concurrent substance use that is exacerbating the condition.

Comorbidity

Systemic hypertension, coronary artery disease, heart failure, stroke, diabetes, and increased mortality are consistently associated with obstructive sleep apnea hypopnea. Risk estimates vary from 30% to as much as 300% for moderate to severe obstructive sleep apnea hypopnea. Evidence of pulmonary hypertension and right heart failure (e.g., cor pulmonale, ankle edema, hepatic congestion) are rare in obstructive sleep apnea hypopnea and when present indicate either very severe disease or associated hypoventilation or cardiopulmonary comorbidities. Obstructive sleep apnea hypopnea also may occur with increased frequency in association with a number of medical or neurological conditions (e.g., cerebrovascular disease, Parkinson's disease). Physical findings reflect the co-occurrence of these conditions.

As many as one-third of individuals referred for evaluation of obstructive sleep apnea hypopnea report symptoms of depression, with as many of 10% having depression scores consistent with moderate to severe depression. Severity of obstructive sleep apnea hypopnea, as measured by the apnea hypopnea index, has been found to be correlated with severity of symptoms of depression. This association may be stronger in males than in females.

Relationship to International Classification of Sleep Disorders

The *International Classification of Sleep Disorders*, 2nd Edition (ICSD-2), differentiates 11 subtypes of "sleep-related breathing disorders," including primary central sleep apnea, obstructive sleep apnea, and sleep-related hypoventilation.

Central Sleep Apnea

Diagnostic Criteria

A. Evidence by polysomnography of five or more central apneas per hour of sleep.

B. The disorder is not better explained by another current sleep disorder.

Specify whether:

327.21 (G47.31) Idiopathic central sleep apnea: Characterized by repeated episodes of apneas and hypopneas during sleep caused by variability in respiratory effort but without evidence of airway obstruction.

786.04 (R06.3) Cheyne-Stokes breathing: A pattern of periodic crescendo-decrescendo variation in tidal volume that results in central apneas and hypopneas at a frequency of at least five events per hour, accompanied by frequent arousal.

780.57 (G47.37) Central sleep apnea comorbid with opioid use: The pathogenesis of this subtype is attributed to the effects of opioids on the respiratory rhythm generators in the medulla as well as the differential effects on hypoxic versus hypercapnic respiratory drive.

Coding note (for 780.57 [G47.37] code only): When an opioid use disorder is present, first code the opioid use disorder: 305.50 (F11.10) mild opioid use disorder or 304.00 (F11.20) moderate or severe opioid use disorder; then code 780.57 (G47.37) central sleep apnea comorbid with opioid use. When an opioid use disorder is not present (e.g., after a one-time heavy use of the substance), code only 780.57 (G47.37) central sleep apnea comorbid with opioid use.

Note: See the section "Diagnostic Features" in text.

Specify current severity:

Severity of central sleep apnea is graded according to the frequency of the breathing disturbances as well as the extent of associated oxygen desaturation and sleep fragmentation that occur as a consequence of repetitive respiratory disturbances.

Subtypes

Idiopathic central sleep apnea and Cheyne-Stokes breathing are characterized by increased gain of the ventilatory control system, also referred to as *high loop gain,* which leads to instability in ventilation and $PaCO_2$ levels. This instability is termed *periodic breathing* and can be recognized by hyperventilation alternating with hypoventilation. Individuals with these disorders typically have pCO_2 levels while awake that are slightly hypocapneic or normocapneic. Central sleep apnea may also manifest during initiation of treatment of obstructive sleep apnea hypopnea or may occur in association with obstructive sleep apnea hypopnea syndrome (termed *complex sleep apnea*). The occurrence of central sleep apnea in association with obstructive sleep apnea is also considered to be due to high loop gain. In contrast, the pathogenesis of central sleep apnea comorbid with opioid use has been attributed to the effects of opioids on the respiratory rhythm generators in the medulla as well as to its differential effects on hypoxic versus hypercapneic respiratory drive. These individuals may have elevated pCO_2 levels while awake. Individuals receiving chronic methadone maintenance therapy have been noted to have increased somnolence and depression, although the role of breathing disorders associated with opioid medication in causing these problems has not been studied.

Specifiers

An increase in the central apnea index (i.e., number of central apneas per hour of sleep) reflects an increase in severity of central sleep apnea. Sleep continuity and quality may be markedly impaired with reductions in restorative stages of non–rapid eye movement (REM) sleep (i.e., decreased slow-wave sleep [stage N3]). In individuals with severe Cheyne-Stokes breathing, the pattern can also be observed during resting wakefulness, a finding that is thought to be a poor prognostic marker for mortality.

Diagnostic Features

Central sleep apnea disorders are characterized by repeated episodes of apneas and hypopneas during sleep caused by variability in respiratory effort. These are disorders of ventilatory control in which respiratory events occur in a periodic or intermittent pattern. *Idiopathic central sleep apnea* is characterized by sleepiness, insomnia, and awakenings due to dyspnea in association with five or more central apneas per hour of sleep. Central sleep apnea occurring in individuals with heart failure, stroke, or renal failure typically have a breathing pattern called *Cheyne-Stokes breathing,* which is characterized by a pattern of periodic crescendo-decrescendo variation in tidal volume that results in central apneas and hypopneas occurring at a frequency of at least five events per hour that are accompanied by frequent arousals. Central and obstructive sleep apneas may coexist; the ratio of central to obstructive apneas/hypopneas may be used to identify which condition is predominant.

Alterations in neuromuscular control of breathing can occur in association with medications or substances used in individuals with mental health conditions, which can cause or exacerbate impairments of respiratory rhythm and ventilation. Individuals taking these medications have a sleep-related breathing disorder that could contribute to sleep disturbances and symptoms such as sleepiness, confusion, and depression. Specifically, *chronic use of long-acting opioid medications* is often associated with impairment of respiratory control leading to central sleep apnea.

Associated Features Supporting Diagnosis

Individuals with central sleep apnea hypopneas can manifest with sleepiness or insomnia. There can be complaints of sleep fragmentation, including awakening with dyspnea. Some individuals are asymptomatic. Obstructive sleep apnea hypopnea can coexist with Cheyne-Stokes breathing, and thus snoring and abruptly terminating apneas may be observed during sleep.

Prevalence

The prevalence of idiopathic central sleep apnea is unknown but thought to be rare. The prevalence of Cheyne-Stokes breathing is high in individuals with depressed cardiac ventricular ejection fraction. In individuals with an ejection fraction of less than 45%, the prevalence has been reported to be 20% or higher. The male-to-female ratio for prevalence is even more highly skewed toward males than for obstructive sleep apnea hypopnea. Prevalence increases with age, and most patients are older than 60 years. Cheyne-Stokes breathing occurs in approximately 20% of individuals with acute stroke. Central sleep apnea comorbid with opioid use occurs in approximately 30% of individuals taking chronic opioids for nonmalignant pain and similarly in individuals receiving methadone maintenance therapy.

Development and Course

The onset of Cheyne-Stokes breathing appears tied to the development of heart failure. The Cheyne-Stokes breathing pattern is associated with oscillations in heart rate, blood pressure and oxygen desaturation, and elevated sympathetic nervous system activity that can promote progression of heart failure. The clinical significance of Cheyne-Stokes breathing in the setting of stroke is not known, but Cheyne-Stokes breathing may be a transient finding that resolves with time after acute stroke. Central sleep apnea comorbid with opioid use has been documented with chronic use (i.e., several months).

Risk and Prognostic Factors

Genetic and physiological.   Cheyne-Stokes breathing is frequently present in individuals with heart failure. The coexistence of atrial fibrillation further increases risk, as do older age and male gender. Cheyne-Stokes breathing is also seen in association with acute stroke and possibly renal failure. The underlying ventilatory instability in the setting of heart failure has been attributed to increased ventilatory chemosensitivity and hyperventilation due to pulmonary vascular congestion and circulatory delay. Central sleep apnea is seen in individuals taking long-acting opioids.

Diagnostic Markers

Physical findings seen in individuals with a Cheyne-Stokes breathing pattern relate to its risk factors. Findings consistent with heart failure, such as jugular venous distension, S_3 heart sound, lung crackles, and lower extremity edema, may be present. Polysomnography is used to characterize the breathing characteristics of each breathing-related sleep disorder subtype. Central sleep apneas are recorded when periods of breathing cessation for longer than 10 seconds occur. Cheyne-Stokes breathing is characterized by a pattern of periodic crescendo-decrescendo variation in tidal volume that results in central apneas and hypopneas occurring at a frequency of at least five events per hour that are accompanied by frequent arousals. The cycle length of Cheyne-Stokes breathing (or time from end of one central apnea to the end of the next apnea) is about 60 seconds.

Functional Consequences of Central Sleep Apnea

Idiopathic central sleep apnea has been reported to cause symptoms of disrupted sleep, including insomnia and sleepiness. Cheyne-Stokes breathing with comorbid heart failure has been associated with excessive sleepiness, fatigue, and insomnia, although many individuals may be asymptomatic. Coexistence of heart failure and Cheyne-Stokes breathing may be associated with increased cardiac arrhythmias and increased mortality or cardiac transplantation. Individuals with central sleep apnea comorbid with opioid use may present with symptoms of sleepiness or insomnia.

Differential Diagnosis

Idiopathic central sleep apnea must be distinguished from other breathing-related sleep disorders, other sleep disorders, and medical conditions and mental disorders that cause sleep fragmentation, sleepiness, and fatigue. This is achieved using polysomnography.

Other breathing-related sleep disorders and sleep disorders. Central sleep apnea can be distinguished from obstructive sleep apnea hypopnea by the presence of at least five central apneas per hour of sleep. These conditions may co-occur, but central sleep apnea is considered to predominate when the ratio of central to obstructive respiratory events exceeds 50%.

Cheyne-Stokes breathing can be distinguished from other mental disorders, including other sleep disorders, and other medical conditions that cause sleep fragmentation, sleepiness, and fatigue based on the presence of a predisposing condition (e.g., heart failure or stroke) and signs and polysomnographic evidence of the characteristic breathing pattern. Polysomnographic respiratory findings can help distinguish Cheyne-Stokes breathing from insomnia due to other medical conditions. High-altitude periodic breathing has a pattern that resembles Cheyne-Stokes breathing but has a shorter cycle time, occurs only at high altitude, and is not associated with heart failure.

Central sleep apnea comorbid with opioid use can be differentiated from other types of breathing-related sleep disorders based on the use of long-acting opioid medications in conjunction with polysomnographic evidence of central apneas and periodic or ataxic breathing. It can be distinguished from insomnia due to drug or substance use based on polysomnographic evidence of central sleep apnea.

Comorbidity

Central sleep apnea disorders are frequently present in users of long-acting opioids, such as methadone. Individuals taking these medications have a sleep-related breathing disorder that could contribute to sleep disturbances and symptoms such as sleepiness, confusion, and depression. While the individual is asleep, breathing patterns such as central apneas, periodic apneas, and ataxic breathing may be observed. Obstructive sleep apnea hypopnea may coexist with central sleep apnea, and features consistent with this condition can also be present (see "Obstructive Sleep Apnea Hypopnea" earlier in this chapter). Cheyne-Stokes breathing is more commonly observed in association with conditions that include heart failure, stroke, and renal failure and is seen more frequently in individuals with atrial fibrillation. Individuals with Cheyne-Stokes breathing are more likely to be older, to be male, and to have lower weight than individuals with obstructive sleep apnea hypopnea.

Sleep-Related Hypoventilation

Diagnostic Criteria

A. Polysomnograpy demonstrates episodes of decreased respiration associated with elevated CO_2 levels. (**Note:** In the absence of objective measurement of CO_2, persistent low levels of hemoglobin oxygen saturation unassociated with apneic/hypopneic events may indicate hypoventilation.)

B. The disturbance is not better explained by another current sleep disorder.

Specify whether:

327.24 (G47.34) Idiopathic hypoventilation: This subtype is not attributable to any readily identified condition.

327.25 (G47.35) Congenital central alveolar hypoventilation: This subtype is a rare congenital disorder in which the individual typically presents in the perinatal period with shallow breathing, or cyanosis and apnea during sleep.

327.26 (G47.36) Comorbid sleep-related hypoventilation: This subtype occurs as a consequence of a medical condition, such as a pulmonary disorder (e.g., interstitial lung disease, chronic obstructive pulmonary disease) or a neuromuscular or chest wall disorder (e.g., muscular dystrophies, postpolio syndrome, cervical spinal cord injury, kyphoscoliosis), or medications (e.g., benzodiazepines, opiates). It also occurs with obesity (obesity hypoventilation disorder), where it reflects a combination of increased work of breathing due to reduced chest wall compliance and ventilation-perfusion mismatch and variably reduced ventilatory drive. Such individuals usually are characterized by body mass index of greater than 30 and hypercapnia during wakefulness (with a pCO_2 of greater than 45), without other evidence of hypoventilation.

Specify current severity:

Severity is graded according to the degree of hypoxemia and hypercarbia present during sleep and evidence of end organ impairment due to these abnormalities (e.g., right-sided heart failure). The presence of blood gas abnormalities during wakefulness is an indicator of greater severity.

Subtypes

Regarding obesity hypoventilation disorder, the prevalence of obesity hypoventilation in the general population is not known but is thought to be increasing in association with the increased prevalence of obesity and extreme obesity.

Diagnostic Features

Sleep-related hypoventilation can occur independently or, more frequently, comorbid with medical or neurological disorders, medication use, or substance use disorder. Although symptoms are not mandatory to make this diagnosis, individuals often report excessive daytime sleepiness, frequent arousals and awakenings during sleep, morning headaches, and insomnia complaints.

Associated Features Supporting Diagnosis

Individuals with sleep-related hypoventilation can present with sleep-related complaints of insomnia or sleepiness. Episodes of orthopnea can occur in individuals with diaphragm weakness. Headaches upon awakening may be present. During sleep, episodes of shallow breathing may be observed, and obstructive sleep apnea hypopnea or central sleep apnea may coexist. Consequences of ventilatory insufficiency, including pulmonary hypertension, cor pulmonale (right heart failure), polycythemia, and neurocognitive dysfunction, can be present. With progression of ventilatory insufficiency, blood gas abnormalities extend into wakefulness. Features of the medical condition causing sleep-related hypoventilation can also be present. Episodes of hypoventilation may be associated with frequent arousals or bradytachycardia. Individuals may complain of excessive sleepiness and insomnia or morning headaches or may present with findings of neurocognitive dysfunction or depression. Hypoventilation may not be present during wakefulness.

Prevalence

Idiopathic sleep-related hypoventilation in adults is very uncommon. The prevalence of congenital central alveolar hypoventilation is unknown, but the disorder is rare. Comorbid sleep-related hypoventilation (i.e., hypoventilation comorbid with other conditions, such as chronic obstructive pulmonary disease [COPD], neuromuscular disorders, or obesity) is more common.

Development and Course

Idiopathic sleep-related hypoventilation is thought to be a slowly progressive disorder of respiratory impairment. When this disorder occurs comorbidly with other disorders (e.g., COPD, neuromuscular disorders, obesity), disease severity reflects the severity of the underlying condition, and the disorder progresses as the condition worsens. Complications such as pulmonary hypertension, cor pulmonale, cardiac dysrhythmias, polycythemia, neurocognitive dysfunction, and worsening respiratory failure can develop with increasing severity of blood gas abnormalities.

Congenital central alveolar hypoventilation usually manifests at birth with shallow, erratic, or absent breathing. This disorder can also manifest during infancy, childhood, and adulthood because of variable penetrance of the *PHOX2B* mutation. Children with congenital central alveolar hypoventilation are more likely to have disorders of the autonomic nervous system, Hirschsprung's disease, neural crest tumors, and characteristic box-shaped face (i.e., the face is short relative to its width).

Risk and Prognostic Factors

Environmental.   Ventilatory drive can be reduced in individuals using central nervous system depressants, including benzodiazepines, opiates, and alcohol.

Genetic and physiological.   Idiopathic sleep-related hypoventilation is associated with reduced ventilatory drive due to a blunted chemoresponsiveness to CO_2 (reduced respiratory drive; i.e., "won't breathe"), reflecting underlying neurological deficits in centers governing the control of ventilation. More commonly, sleep-related hypoventilation is comorbid with another medical condition, such as a pulmonary disorder, a neuromuscular or chest wall disorder, or hypothyroidism, or with use of medications (e.g., benzodiazepines, opiates). In these conditions, the hypoventilation may be a consequence of increased work of breathing and/or impairment of respiratory muscle function (i.e., "can't breathe") or reduced respiratory drive (i.e., "won't breathe").

Neuromuscular disorders influence breathing through impairment of respiratory motor innervation or respiratory muscle function. They include conditions such as amyotrophic lateral sclerosis, spinal cord injury, diaphragmatic paralysis, myasthenia gravis, Lambert-Eaton syndrome, toxic or metabolic myopathies, postpolio syndrome, and Charcot-Marie-Tooth syndrome.

Congenital central alveolar hypoventilation is a genetic disorder attributable to mutations of *PHOX2B,* a gene that is crucial for the development of the embryonic autonomic nervous system and neural crest derivatives. Children with congenital central alveolar hypoventilation show blunted ventilatory responses to hypercapnia, especially in non–rapid eye movement sleep.

Gender-Related Diagnostic Issues

Gender distributions for sleep-related hypoventilation occurring in association with comorbid conditions reflect the gender distributions of the comorbid conditions. For example, COPD is more frequently present in males and with increasing age.

Diagnostic Markers

Sleep-related hypoventilation is diagnosed using polysomnography showing sleep-related hypoxemia and hypercapnia that is not better explained by another breathing-related sleep disorder. The documentation of increased arterial pCO_2 levels to greater than 55 mmHg during sleep or a 10 mmHg or greater increase in pCO_2 levels (to a level that also exceeds 50 mmHg) during sleep in comparison to awake supine values, for 10 minutes or longer, is the gold standard for diagnosis. However, obtaining arterial blood gas determinations during sleep is impractical, and non-invasive measures of pCO_2 have not been adequately validated during sleep and are not widely used during polysomnography in adults. Prolonged and sustained decreases in oxygen saturation (oxygen saturation of less than 90% for more than 5 minutes with a nadir of at least 85%, or oxygen saturation of less than 90% for at least 30% of sleep time) in the absence of evidence of upper airway obstruction are often used as an indication of sleep-related hypoventilation; however, this finding is not specific, as there are other potential causes of hypoxemia, such as that due to lung disease.

Functional Consequences of Sleep-Related Hypoventilation

The consequences of sleep-related hypoventilation are related to the effects of chronic exposure to hypercapnia and hypoxemia. These blood gas derangements cause vasoconstriction of the pulmonary vasculature leading to pulmonary hypertension, which, if severe, can result in right-sided heart failure (cor pulmonale). Hypoxemia can lead to dysfunction of organs such as the brain, blood, and heart, leading to outcomes such as cognitive dysfunction, polycythemia, and cardiac arrhythmias. Hypercapnia can depress ventilatory drive, leading to progressive respiratory failure.

Differential Diagnosis

Other medical conditions affecting ventilation. In adults, the idiopathic variety of sleep-related hypoventilation is very uncommon and is determined by excluding the presence of lung diseases, skeletal malformations, neuromuscular disorders, and other medical and neurological disorders or medications that affect ventilation. Sleep-related hypoventilation must be distinguished from other causes of sleep-related hypoxemia, such as that due to lung disease.

Other breathing-related sleep disorders. Sleep-related hypoventilation can be distinguished from obstructive sleep apnea hypopnea and central sleep apnea based on clinical features and findings on polysomnography. Sleep-related hypoventilation typically shows more sustained periods of oxygen desaturation rather that the periodic episodes seen in obstructive sleep apnea hypopnea and central sleep apnea. Obstructive sleep apnea hypopnea and central sleep apnea also show a pattern of discrete episodes of repeated airflow decreases that can be absent in sleep-related hypoventilation.

Comorbidity

Sleep-related hypoventilation often occurs in association with a pulmonary disorder (e.g., interstitial lung disease, COPD), with a neuromuscular or chest wall disorder (e.g., muscular dystrophies, post-polio syndrome, cervical spinal cord injury, obesity, kyphoscoliosis), or, most relevant to the mental health provider, with medication use (e.g., benzodiazepines, opiates). Congenital central alveolar hypoventilation often occurs in association with autonomic dysfunction and may occur in association with Hirschsprung's disease. COPD, a disorder of lower airway obstruction usually associated with cigarette smoking, can result in sleep-related hypoventilation and hypoxemia. The presence of coexisting obstructive sleep apnea hypopnea is thought to exacerbate hypoxemia and hypercapnia during sleep and wakefulness. The relationship between congenital central alveolar hypoventilation and idiopathic sleep-related hypoventilation is unclear; in some individuals, idiopathic sleep-related hypoventilation may represent cases of late-onset congenital central alveolar hypoventilation.

Relationship to International Classification of Sleep Disorders

The *International Classification of Sleep Disorders*, 2nd Edition (ICSD-2), combines sleep-related hypoventilation and sleep-related hypoxemia under the category of sleep-related hypoventilation/hypoxemic syndromes. This approach to classification reflects the frequent co-occurrence of disorders that lead to hypoventilation and hypoxemia. In contrast, the classification used in DSM-5 reflects evidence that there are distinct sleep-related pathogenetic processes leading to hypoventilation.

Circadian Rhythm Sleep-Wake Disorders

Diagnostic Criteria

A. A persistent or recurrent pattern of sleep disruption that is primarily due to an alteration of the circadian system or to a misalignment between the endogenous circadian rhythm and the sleep–wake schedule required by an individual's physical environment or social or professional schedule.

B. The sleep disruption leads to excessive sleepiness or insomnia, or both.

C. The sleep disturbance causes clinically significant distress or impairment in social, occupational, and other important areas of functioning.

Coding note: For ICD-9-CM, code **307.45** for all subtypes. For ICD-10-CM, code is based on subtype.

Specify whether:

307.45 (G47.21) Delayed sleep phase type: A pattern of delayed sleep onset and awakening times, with an inability to fall asleep and awaken at a desired or conventionally acceptable earlier time.

> *Specify* if:
> **Familial:** A family history of delayed sleep phase is present.

> *Specify* if:
> **Overlapping with non-24-hour sleep-wake type:** Delayed sleep phase type may overlap with another circadian rhythm sleep-wake disorder, non-24-hour sleep-wake type.

307.45 (G47.22) Advanced sleep phase type: A pattern of advanced sleep onset and awakening times, with an inability to remain awake or asleep until the desired or conventionally acceptable later sleep or wake times.

> *Specify* if:
> **Familial:** A family history of advanced sleep phase is present.

307.45 (G47.23) Irregular sleep-wake type: A temporally disorganized sleep-wake pattern, such that the timing of sleep and wake periods is variable throughout the 24-hour period.

307.45 (G47.24) Non-24-hour sleep-wake type: A pattern of sleep-wake cycles that is not synchronized to the 24-hour environment, with a consistent daily drift (usually to later and later times) of sleep onset and wake times.

307.45 (G47.26) Shift work type: Insomnia during the major sleep period and/or excessive sleepiness (including inadvertent sleep) during the major awake period associated with a shift work schedule (i.e., requiring unconventional work hours).

307.45 (G47.20) Unspecified type

Specify if:
    Episodic: Symptoms last at least 1 month but less than 3 months.
    Persistent: Symptoms last 3 months or longer.
    Recurrent: Two or more episodes occur within the space of 1 year.

Delayed Sleep Phase Type

Diagnostic Features

The delayed sleep phase type is based primarily on a history of a delay in the timing of the major sleep period (usually more than 2 hours) in relation to the desired sleep and wake-up time, resulting in symptoms of insomnia and excessive sleepiness. When allowed to set their own schedule, individuals with delayed sleep phase type exhibit normal sleep quality and duration for age. Symptoms of sleep-onset insomnia, difficulty waking in the morning, and excessive early day sleepiness are prominent.

Associated Features Supporting Diagnosis

Common associated features of delayed sleep phase type include a history of mental disorders or a concurrent mental disorder. Extreme and prolonged difficulty awakening with morning confusion is also common. Psychophysiological insomnia may develop as a result of maladaptive behaviors that impair sleep and increase arousal because of repeated attempts to fall asleep at an earlier time.

Prevalence

Prevalence of delayed sleep phase type in the general population is approximately 0.17% but appears to be greater than 7% in adolescents. Although the prevalence of familial delayed sleep phase type has not been established, a family history of delayed sleep phase is present in individuals with delayed sleep phase type.

Development and Course

Course is persistent, lasting longer than 3 months, with intermittent exacerbations throughout adulthood. Although age at onset is variable, symptoms begin typically in adolescence and early adulthood and persist for several months to years before diagnosis is established. Severity may decrease with age. Relapse of symptoms is common.

Clinical expression may vary across the lifespan depending on social, school, and work obligations. Exacerbation is usually triggered by a change in work or school schedule that requires an early rise time. Individuals who can alter their work schedules to accommodate the delayed circadian sleep and wake timing can experience remission of symptoms.

Increased prevalence in adolescence may be a consequence of both physiological and behavioral factors. Hormonal changes may be involved specifically, as delayed sleep phase is associated with the onset of puberty. Thus, delayed sleep phase type in adolescents should be differentiated from the common delay in the timing of circadian rhythms in this age group. In the familial form, the course is persistent and may not improve significantly with age.

Risk and Prognostic Factors

Genetic and physiological.   Predisposing factors may include a longer than average circadian period, changes in light sensitivity, and impaired homeostatic sleep drive. Some individuals with delayed sleep phase type may be hypersensitive to evening light, which can serve as a delay signal to the circadian clock, or they may be hyposensitive to morning light such that its phase-advancing effects are reduced. Genetic factors may play a role in the pathogenesis of familial and sporadic forms of delayed sleep phase type, including mutations in circadian genes (e.g., *PER3*, *CKIe*).

Diagnostic Markers

Confirmation of the diagnosis includes a complete history and use of a sleep diary or actigraphy (i.e., a wrist-worn motion detector that monitors motor activity for prolonged periods and can be used as a proxy for sleep-wake patterns for at least 7 days). The period covered should include weekends, when social and occupational obligations are less strict, to ensure that the individual exhibits a consistently delayed sleep-wake pattern. Biomarkers such as salivary dim light melatonin onset should be obtained only when the diagnosis is unclear.

Functional Consequences of Delayed Sleep Phase Type

Excessive early day sleepiness is prominent. Extreme and prolonged difficulty awakening with morning confusion (i.e., sleep inertia) is also common. The severity of insomnia and excessive sleepiness symptoms varies substantially among individuals and largely depends on the occupational and social demands on the individual.

Differential Diagnosis

Normative variations in sleep.   Delayed sleep phase type must be distinguished from "normal" sleep patterns in which an individual has a late schedule that does not cause personal, social, or occupational distress (most commonly seen in adolescents and young adults).

Other sleep disorders.   Insomnia disorder and other circadian rhythm sleep-wake disorders should be included in the differential. Excessive sleepiness may also be caused by other sleep disturbances, such as breathing-related sleep disorders, insomnias, sleep-related movement disorders, and medical, neurological, and mental disorders. Overnight polysomnography may help in evaluating for other comorbid sleep disorders, such as sleep apnea. The circadian nature of delayed sleep phase type, however, should differentiate it from other disorders with similar complaints.

Comorbidity

Delayed sleep phase type is strongly associated with depression, personality disorder, and somatic symptom disorder or illness anxiety disorder. In addition, comorbid sleep disorders, such as insomnia disorder, restless legs syndrome, and sleep apnea, as well as depressive and bipolar disorders and anxiety disorders, can exacerbate symptoms of insomnia and excessive sleepiness. Delayed sleep phase type may overlap with another circadian rhythm sleep-wake disorder, non-24-hour sleep-wake type. Sighted individuals with non-24-hour sleep-wake type disorder commonly also have a history of delayed circadian sleep phase.

Advanced Sleep Phase Type

Specifiers

Advanced sleep phase type may be documented with the specified "familial." Although the prevalence of familial advanced sleep phase type has not been established, a family history of advanced sleep phase is present in individuals with advanced sleep phase type. In this type, specific mutations demonstrate an autosomal dominant mode of inheritance. In the familial form, onset of symptoms may occur earlier (during childhood and early adulthood), the course is persistent, and the severity of symptoms may increase with age.

Diagnostic Features

Advanced sleep phase type is characterized by sleep-wake times that are several hours earlier than desired or conventional times. Diagnosis is based primarily on a history of an advance in the timing of the major sleep period (usually more than 2 hours) in relation to the desired sleep and wake-up time, with symptoms of early morning insomnia and excessive daytime sleepiness. When allowed to set their schedule, individuals with advanced sleep phase type will exhibit normal sleep quality and duration for age.

Associated Features Supporting Diagnosis

Individuals with advanced sleep phase type are "morning types," having earlier sleep-wake times, with the timing of circadian biomarkers such as melatonin and core body temperature rhythms occurring 2–4 hours earlier than normal. When required to keep a conventional schedule requiring a delay of bedtime, these individuals will continue to have an early rise time, leading to persistent sleep deprivation and daytime sleepiness. Use of hypnotics or alcohol to combat sleep-maintenance insomnia and stimulants to reduce daytime sleepiness may lead to substance abuse in these individuals.

Prevalence

The estimated prevalence of advanced sleep phase type is approximately 1% in middle-age adults. Sleep-wake times and circadian phase advance in older individuals, probably accounting for increased prevalence in this population.

Development and Course

Onset is usually in late adulthood. In the familial form, onset can be earlier. The course is typically persistent, lasting more than 3 months, but the severity may increase depending on work and social schedules. The advanced sleep phase type is more common in older adults.

Clinical expression may vary across the lifespan depending on social, school, and work obligations. Individuals who can alter their work schedules to accommodate the advanced circadian sleep and wake timing can experience remission of symptoms. Increasing age tends to advance the sleep phase, however, it is unclear whether the common age-associated advanced sleep phase type is due solely to a change in circadian timing (as seen in the familial form) or also to age-related changes in the homeostatic regulation of sleep, resulting in earlier awakening. Severity, remission, and relapse of symptoms suggest lack of adherence to behavioral and environmental treatments designed to control sleep and wake structure and light exposure.

Risk and Prognostic Factors

Environmental.   Decreased late afternoon/early evening exposure to light and/or exposure to early morning light due to early morning awakening can increase the risk of advanced sleep phase type by advancing circadian rhythms. By going to bed early, these individuals are not exposed to light in the phase delay region of the curve, resulting in perpetuation of advanced phase. In familial advanced sleep phase type, a shortening of the endogenous circadian period can result in an advanced sleep phase, although circadian period does not appear to systematically decrease with age.

Genetic and physiological.   Advanced sleep phase type has demonstrated an autosomal dominant mode of inheritance, including a *PER2* gene mutation causing hypophosphorylation of the PER2 protein and a missense mutation in *CKI*.

Culture-Related Diagnostic Issues

African Americans may have a shorter circadian period and larger magnitude phase advances to light than do Caucasians, possibly increasing the risk for development of advanced sleep phase type in this population.

Diagnostic Markers

A sleep diary and actigraphy may be used as diagnostic markers, as described earlier for delayed sleep phase type.

Functional Consequences of Advanced Sleep Phase Type

Excessive sleepiness associated with advanced sleep phase can have a negative effect on cognitive performance, social interaction, and safety. Use of wake-promoting agents to combat sleepiness or sedatives for early morning awakening may increase potential for substance abuse.

Differential Diagnosis

Other sleep disorders.   Behavioral factors such as irregular sleep schedules, voluntary early awakening, and exposure to light in the early morning should be considered, particularly in older adults. Careful attention should be paid to rule out other sleep-wake disorders, such as insomnia disorder, and other mental disorders and medical conditions that can cause early morning awakening.

Depressive and bipolar disorders. Because early morning awakening, fatigue, and sleepiness are prominent features of major depressive disorder, depressive and bipolar disorders must also be considered.

Comorbidity

Medical conditions and mental disorders with the symptom of early morning awakening, such as insomnia, can co-occur with the advance sleep phase type.

Irregular Sleep-Wake Type

Diagnostic Features

The diagnosis of irregular sleep-wake type is based primarily on a history of symptoms of insomnia at night (during the usual sleep period) and excessive sleepiness (napping) during the day. Irregular sleep-wake type is characterized by a lack of discernable sleep-wake circadian rhythm. There is no major sleep period, and sleep is fragmented into at least three periods during the 24-hour day.

Associated Features Supporting Diagnosis

Individuals with irregular sleep-wake type typically present with insomnia or excessive sleepiness, depending on the time of day. Sleep and wake periods across 24 hours are fragmented, although the longest sleep period tends to occur between 2:00 A.M. and 6:00 A.M. and is usually less than 4 hours. A history of isolation or reclusion may occur in association with the disorder and contribute to the symptoms via a lack of external stimuli to help entrain a normal pattern. Individuals or their caregivers report frequent naps throughout the day. Irregular sleep-wake type is most commonly associated with neurodegenerative disorders, such as major neurocognitive disorder, and many neurodevelopmental disorders in children.

Prevalence

Prevalence of irregular sleep-wake type in the general population is unknown.

Development and Course

The course of irregular sleep-wake type is persistent. Age at onset is variable, but the disorder is more common in older adults.

Risk and Prognostic Factors

Temperamental. Neurodegenerative disorders, such as Alzheimer's disease, Parkinson's disease, and Huntington's disease, and neurodevelopmental disorders in children increase the risk for irregular sleep-wake type.

Environmental. Decreased exposure to environmental light and structured daytime activity can be associated with a low-amplitude circadian rhythm. Hospitalized individuals are especially prone to such weak external entraining stimuli, and even outside the hospital setting, individuals with major neurocognitive disorder (i.e., dementia) are exposed to significantly less bright light.

Diagnostic Markers

A detailed sleep history and a sleep diary (by a caregiver) or actigraphy help confirm the irregular sleep-wake pattern.

Functional Consequences of Irregular Sleep-Wake Type

Lack of a clearly discernible major sleep and wake period in irregular sleep-wake type results in insomnia or excessive sleepiness, depending on the time of day. Disruption of the caregiver's sleep also often occurs and is an important consideration.

Differential Diagnosis

Normative variations in sleep.   Irregular sleep-wake type should be distinguished from a voluntary irregular sleep-wake schedule and poor sleep hygiene, which can result in insomnia and excessive sleepiness.

Other medical conditions and mental disorders.   Other causes of insomnia and daytime sleepiness, including comorbid medical conditions and mental disorders or medication, should be considered.

Comorbidity

Irregular sleep-wake type is often comorbid with neurodegenerative and neurodevelopmental disorders, such as major neurocognitive disorder, intellectual disability (intellectual developmental disorder), and traumatic brain injury. It is also comorbid with other medical conditions and mental disorders in which there is social isolation and/or lack of light and structured activities.

Non-24-Hour Sleep-Wake Type

Diagnostic Features

The diagnosis of non-24-hour sleep-wake type is based primarily on a history of symptoms of insomnia or excessive sleepiness related to abnormal synchronization between the 24-hour light-dark cycle and the endogenous circadian rhythm. Individuals typically present with periods of insomnia, excessive sleepiness, or both, which alternate with short asymptomatic periods. Starting with the asymptomatic period, when the individual's sleep phase is aligned to the external environment, sleep latency will gradually increase and the individual will complain of sleep-onset insomnia. As the sleep phase continues to drift so that sleep time is now in the daytime, the individual will have trouble staying awake during the day and will complain of sleepiness. Because the circadian period is not aligned to the external 24-hour environment, symptoms will depend on when an individual tries to sleep in relation to the circadian rhythm of sleep propensity.

Associated Features Supporting Diagnosis

Non-24-hour sleep-wake type is most common among blind or visually impaired individuals who have decreased light perception. In sighted individuals, there is often a history of delayed sleep phase and of decreased exposure to light and structured social and physical activity. Sighted individuals with non-24-hour sleep-wake type also demonstrate increased sleep duration.

Prevalence

Prevalence of non-24-hour sleep-wake type in the general population is unclear, but the disorder appears rare in sighted individuals. The prevalence in blind individuals is estimated to be 50%.

Development and Course

Course of non-24-hour sleep-wake type is persistent, with intermittent remission and exacerbations due to changes in work and social schedules throughout the lifespan. Age at onset is variable, depending on the onset of visual impairment. In sighted individuals, because of the overlap with delayed sleep phase type, non-24-hour sleep-wake type may develop in adolescence or early adulthood. Remission and relapse of symptoms in blind and sighted individuals largely depend on adherence to treatments designed to control sleep and wake structure and light exposure.

Clinical expression may vary across the lifespan depending on social, school, and work obligations. In adolescents and adults, irregular sleep-wake schedules and exposure to light or lack of light at critical times of the day can exacerbate the effects of sleep loss and disrupt circadian entrainment. Consequently, symptoms of insomnia, daytime sleepiness, and school, professional, and interpersonal functioning may worsen.

Risk and Prognostic Factors

Environmental. In sighted individuals, decreased exposure or sensitivity to light and social and physical activity cues may contribute to a free-running circadian rhythm. With the high frequency of mental disorders involving social isolation and cases of non-24-hour sleep-wake type developing after a change in sleep habits (e.g., night shift work, job loss), behavioral factors in combination with physiological tendency may precipitate and perpetuate this disorder in sighted individuals. Hospitalized individuals with neurological and psychiatric disorders can become insensitive to social cues, predisposing them to the development of non-24-hour sleep-wake type.

Genetic and physiological. Blindness is a risk factor for non-24-hour sleep-wake type. Non-24-hour sleep-wake type has been associated with traumatic brain injury.

Diagnostic Markers

Diagnosis is confirmed by history and sleep diary or actigraphy for an extended period. Sequential measurement of phase markers (e.g., melatonin) can help determine circadian phase in both sighted and blind individuals.

Functional Consequences of Non-24-Hour Sleep-Wake Type

Complaints of insomnia (sleep onset and sleep maintenance), excessive sleepiness, or both are prominent. The unpredictability of sleep and wake times (typically a daily delay drift) results in an inability to attend school or maintain a steady job and may increase potential for social isolation.

Differential Diagnosis

Circadian rhythm sleep-wake disorders.   In sighted individuals, non-24-hour sleep-wake type should be differentiated from delayed sleep phase type, as individuals with delayed sleep phase type may display a similar progressive delay in sleep period for several days.

Depressive disorders.   Depressive symptoms and depressive disorders may result in similar circadian dysregulation and symptoms.

Comorbidity

Blindness is often comorbid with non-24-hour sleep-wake type, as are depressive and bipolar disorders with social isolation.

Shift Work Type

Diagnostic Features

Diagnosis is primarily based on a history of the individual working outside of the normal 8:00 A.M. to 6:00 P.M. daytime window (particularly at night) on a regularly scheduled (i.e., non-overtime) basis. Symptoms of excessive sleepiness at work, and impaired sleep at home, on a persistent basis are prominent. Presence of both sets of symptoms are usually required for a diagnosis of shift work type. Typically, when the individual reverts to a day-work routine, symptoms resolve. Although the etiology is slightly different, individuals who travel across many time zones on a very frequent basis may experience effects similar to those experienced by individuals with shift work type who work rotating shifts.

Prevalence

The prevalence of shift work type is unclear, but the disorder is estimated to affect 5%–10% of the night worker population (16%–20% of the workforce). Prevalence rises with advancement into middle-age and beyond.

Development and Course

Shift work type can appear in individuals of any age but is more prevalent in individuals older than 50 years and typically worsens with the passage of time if the disruptive work hours persist. Although older adults may show similar rates of circadian phase adjustment to a change in routine as do younger adults, they appear to experience significantly more sleep disruption as a consequence of the circadian phase shift.

Risk and Prognostic Factors

Temperamental. Predisposing factors include a morning-type disposition, a need for long (i.e., more than 8 hours) sleep durations in order to feel well rested, and strong competing social and domestic needs (e.g., parents of young children). Individuals who are able to commit to a nocturnal lifestyle, with few competing day-oriented demands, appear at lower risk for shift work type.

Genetic and physiological. Because shift workers are more likely than day workers to be obese, obstructive sleep apnea may be present and may exacerbate the symptoms.

Diagnostic Markers

A history and sleep diary or actigraphy may be useful in diagnosis, as discussed earlier for delayed sleep phase type.

Functional Consequences of Shift Work Type

Individuals with shift work type not only may perform poorly at work but also appear to be at risk for accidents both at work and on the drive home. They may also be at risk for poor mental health (e.g., alcohol use disorder, substance use disorder, depression) and physical health (e.g., gastrointestinal disorders, cardiovascular disease, diabetes, cancer). Individuals with a history of bipolar disorder are particularly vulnerable to shift work type–related episodes of mania resulting from missed nights of sleep. Shift work type often results in interpersonal problems.

Differential Diagnosis

Normative variations in sleep with shift work. The diagnosis of shift work type, as opposed to the "normal" difficulties of shift work, must depend to some extent on the severity of symptoms and/or level of distress experienced by the individual. Presence of shift work type symptoms even when the individual is able to live on a day-oriented routine for several weeks at a time may suggest the presence of other sleep disorders, such as sleep apnea, insomnia, and narcolepsy, which should be ruled out.

Comorbidity

Shift work type has been associated with increased alcohol use disorder, other substance use disorders, and depression. A variety of physical health disorders (e.g., gastrointestinal disorders, cardiovascular disease, diabetes, cancer) have been found to be associated with prolonged exposure to shift work.

Relationship to International Classification of Sleep Disorders

The *International Classification of Sleep Disorders*, 2nd Edition (ICSD-2), differentiates nine circadian rhythm sleep disorders, including jet lag type.

Parasomnias

Parasomnias are disorders characterized by abnormal behavioral, experiential, or physiological events occurring in association with sleep, specific sleep stages, or sleep-wake transitions. The most common parasomnias—non–rapid eye movement (NREM) sleep arousal disorders and rapid eye movement (REM) sleep behavior disorder—represent admixtures of wakefulness and NREM sleep and wakefulness and REM sleep, respectively. These conditions serve as a reminder that sleep and wakefulness are not mutually exclusive and that sleep is not necessarily a global, whole-brain phenomenon.

Non–Rapid Eye Movement Sleep Arousal Disorders

Diagnostic Criteria

A. Recurrent episodes of incomplete awakening from sleep, usually occurring during the first third of the major sleep episode, accompanied by either one of the following:

1. **Sleepwalking:** Repeated episodes of rising from bed during sleep and walking about. While sleepwalking, the individual has a blank, staring face; is relatively unresponsive to the efforts of others to communicate with him or her; and can be awakened only with great difficulty.

2. **Sleep terrors:** Recurrent episodes of abrupt terror arousals from sleep, usually beginning with a panicky scream. There is intense fear and signs of autonomic arousal, such as mydriasis, tachycardia, rapid breathing, and sweating, during each episode. There is relative unresponsiveness to efforts of others to comfort the individual during the episodes.

B. No or little (e.g., only a single visual scene) dream imagery is recalled.

C. Amnesia for the episodes is present.

D. The episodes cause clinically significant distress or impairment in social, occupational, or other important areas of functioning.

E. The disturbance is not attributable to the physiological effects of a substance (e.g., a drug of abuse, a medication).

F. Coexisting mental and medical disorders do not explain the episodes of sleepwalking or sleep terrors.

Coding note: For ICD-9-CM, code **307.46** for all subtypes. For ICD-10-CM, code is based on subtype.

Specify whether:

307.46 (F51.3) Sleepwalking type

Specify if:

With sleep-related eating

With sleep-related sexual behavior (sexsomnia)

307.46 (F51.4) Sleep terror type

Diagnostic Features

The essential feature of non–rapid eye movement (NREM) sleep arousal disorders is the repeated occurrence of incomplete arousals, usually beginning during the first third of the major sleep episode (Criterion A), that typically are brief, lasting 1–10 minutes, but may be protracted, lasting up to 1 hour. The maximum duration of an event is unknown. The eyes are typically open during these events. Many individuals exhibit both subtypes of arousals on different occasions, which underscores the unitary underlying pathophysiology. The subtypes reflect varying degrees of simultaneous occurrence of wakefulness and NREM sleep, resulting in complex behaviors arising from sleep with varying degrees of conscious awareness, motor activity, and autonomic activation.

The essential feature of *sleepwalking* is repeated episodes of complex motor behavior initiated during sleep, including rising from bed and walking about (Criterion A1). Sleepwalking episodes begin during any stage of NREM sleep, most commonly during slow-wave sleep and therefore most often occurring during the first third of the night. During episodes, the individual has reduced alertness and responsiveness, a blank stare, and relative unresponsiveness to communication with others or efforts by others to awaken the individual. If awakened during the episode (or on awakening the following morning), the individual has limited recall for the episode. After the episode, there may initially be a brief period of confusion or difficulty orienting, followed by full recovery of cognitive function and appropriate behavior.

The essential feature of *sleep terrors* is the repeated occurrence of precipitous awakenings from sleep, usually beginning with a panicky scream or cry (Criterion A2). Sleep terrors usually begin during the first third of the major sleep episode and last 1–10 minutes, but they may last considerably longer, particularly in children. The episodes are accompanied by impressive autonomic arousal and behavioral manifestations of intense fear. During an episode, the individual is difficult to awaken or comfort. If the individual awakens after the sleep terror, little or none of the dream, or only fragmentary, single images, are recalled. During a typical episode of sleep terrors, the individual abruptly sits up in bed screaming or crying, with a frightened expression and autonomic signs of intense anxiety (e.g., tachycardia, rapid breathing, sweating, dilation of the pupils). The individual may be inconsolable and is usually unresponsive to the efforts of others to awaken or comfort him or her. Sleep terrors are also called "night terrors" or "pavor nocturnus."

Associated Features Supporting Diagnosis

Sleepwalking episodes can include a wide variety of behaviors. Episodes may begin with confusion: the individual may simply sit up in bed, look about, or pick at the blanket or sheet. This behavior then becomes progressively complex. The individual may actually leave the bed and walk into closets, out of the room, and even out of buildings. Individuals may use the bathroom, eat, talk, or engage in more complex behaviors. Running and frantic attempts to escape some apparent threat can also occur. Most behaviors during sleepwalking episodes are routine and of low complexity. However, cases of unlocking doors and even operating machinery (driving an automobile) have been reported. Sleepwalking can also include inappropriate behavior (e.g., commonly, urinating in a closet or wastebasket). Most episodes last for several minutes to a half hour but may be more protracted. Inasmuch as sleep is a state of relative analgesia, painful injuries sustained during sleepwalking may not be appreciated until awakening after the fact.

There are two "specialized" forms of sleepwalking: sleep-related eating behavior and sleep-related sexual behavior (sexsomnia or sleep sex). Individuals with *sleep-related eating* experience unwanted recurrent episodes of eating with varying degrees of amnesia, ranging from no awareness to full awareness without the ability to not eat. During these episodes, inappropriate foods may be ingested. Individuals with sleep-related eating disorder may find evidence of their eating only the next morning. In *sexsomnia*, varying degrees of sexual activity (e.g., masturbation, fondling, groping, sexual intercourse) occur as complex behaviors arising from sleep without conscious awareness. This condition is more common in males and may result in serious interpersonal relationship problems or medicolegal consequences.

During a typical episode of sleep terrors, there is often a sense of overwhelming dread, with a compulsion to escape. Although fragmentary vivid dream images may occur, a storylike dream sequence (as in nightmares) is not reported. Most commonly, the individual does not awaken fully, but returns to sleep and has amnesia for the episode on awakening the next morning. Usually only one episode will occur on any one night. Occasionally several episodes may occur at intervals throughout the night. These events rarely arise during daytime naps.

Prevalence

Isolated or infrequent NREM sleep arousal disorders are very common in the general population. From 10% to 30% of children have had at least one episode of sleepwalking, and 2%–3% sleepwalk often. The prevalence of sleepwalking disorder, marked by repeated episodes and impairment or distress, is much lower, probably in the range of 1%–5%. The prevalence of sleepwalking episodes (not sleepwalking disorder) is 1.0%–7.0% among adults, with weekly to monthly episodes occurring in 0.5%–0.7%. The lifetime prevalence of sleepwalking in adults is 29.2%, with a past-year prevalence of sleepwalking of 3.6%.

The prevalence of sleep terrors in the general population is unknown. The prevalence of sleep terror episodes (as opposed to sleep terror disorder, in which there is recurrence and distress or impairment) is approximately 36.9% at 18 months of age, 19.7% at 30 months of age, and 2.2% in adults.

Development and Course

NREM sleep arousal disorders occur most commonly in childhood and diminish in frequency with increasing age. The onset of sleepwalking in adults with no prior history of sleepwalking as children should prompt a search for specific etiologies, such as obstructive sleep apnea, nocturnal seizures, or effect of medication.

Risk and Prognostic Factors

Environmental. Sedative use, sleep deprivation, sleep-wake schedule disruptions, fatigue, and physical or emotional stress increase the likelihood of episodes. Fever and sleep deprivation can produce an increased frequency of NREM sleep arousal disorders.

Genetic and physiological. A family history for sleepwalking or sleep terrors may occur in up to 80% of individuals who sleepwalk. The risk for sleepwalking is further increased (to as much as 60% of offspring) when both parents have a history of the disorder.

Individuals with sleep terrors frequently have a positive family history of either sleep terrors or sleepwalking, with as high as a 10-fold increase in the prevalence of the disorder among first-degree biological relatives. Sleep terrors are much more common in monozygotic twins as compared with dizygotic twins. The exact mode of inheritance is unknown.

Gender-Related Diagnostic Issues

Violent or sexual activity during sleepwalking episodes is more likely to occur in adults. Eating during sleepwalking episodes is more commonly seen in females. Sleepwalking occurs more often in females during childhood but more often in males during adulthood.

Older children and adults provide a more detailed recollection of fearful images associated with sleep terrors than do younger children, who are more likely to have complete amnesia or report only a vague sense of fear. Among children, sleep terrors are more common in males than in females. Among adults, the sex ratio is even.

Diagnostic Markers

NREM sleep arousal disorders arise from any stage of NREM sleep but most commonly from deep NREM sleep (slow-wave sleep). They are most likely to appear in the first third of the night and do not commonly occur during daytime naps. During the episode, the polysomnogram may be obscured with movement artifact. In the absence of such artifact, the electroencephalogram typically shows theta or alpha frequency activity during the episode, indicating partial or incomplete arousal.

Polysomnography in conjunction with audiovisual monitoring can be used to document episodes of sleepwalking. In the absence of actually capturing an event during a polysomnographic recording, there are no polysomnographic features that can serve as a marker for sleepwalking. Sleep deprivation may increase the likelihood of capturing an event. As a group, individuals who sleepwalk show instability of deep NREM sleep, but the overlap in findings with individuals who do not sleepwalk is great enough to preclude use of this indicator in establishing a diagnosis. Unlike arousals from REM sleep associated with nightmares, in which there is an increase in heart rate and respiration prior to the arousal, the NREM sleep arousals of sleep terrors begin precipitously from sleep, without anticipatory autonomic changes. The arousals are associated with impressive autonomic activity, with doubling or tripling of the heart rate. The pathophysiology is poorly understood, but there appears to be instability in the deeper stages of NREM sleep. Absent capturing an event during a formal sleep study, there are no reliable polysomnographic indicators of the tendency to experience sleep terrors.

Functional Consequences of Non-REM Sleep Arousal Disorders

For the diagnosis of a NREM sleep arousal disorder to be made, the individual or household members must experience clinically significant distress or impairment, although parasomnia symptoms may occur occasionally in nonclinical populations and would be subthreshold for the diagnosis. Embarrassment concerning the episodes can impair social relationships. Social isolation or occupational difficulties can result. The determination of a "disorder" depends on a number of factors, which may vary on an individual basis and will depend on the frequency of events, potential for violence or injurious behaviors, embarrassment, or disruption/distress of other household members. Severity determination is best made based on the nature or consequence of the behaviors rather than simply on frequency. Uncommonly, NREM sleep arousal disorders may result in serious injury to the individual or to someone trying to console the individual. Injuries to others are confined to those in close proximity; individuals are not "sought out." Typically, sleepwalking in both children and adults is not associated with significant mental disorders. For individuals with sleep-related eating behaviors, unknowingly preparing or eating food during the sleep period may create problems such as poor diabetes control, weight gain, injury (cuts and burns), or consequences of eating dangerous or toxic inedibles. NREM sleep arousal disorders may rarely result in violent or injurious behaviors with forensic implications.

Differential Diagnosis

Nightmare disorder.   In contrast to individuals with NREM sleep arousal disorders, individuals with nightmare disorder typically awaken easily and completely, report vivid storylike dreams accompanying the episodes, and tend to have episodes later in the night. NREM sleep arousal disorders occur during NREM sleep, whereas nightmares usually occur during REM sleep. Parents of children with NREM sleep arousal disorders may misinterpret reports of fragmentary imagery as nightmares.

Breathing-related sleep disorders.   Breathing disorders during sleep can also produce confusional arousals with subsequent amnesia. However, breathing-related sleep disorders are also characterized by characteristic symptoms of snoring, breathing pauses, and daytime sleepiness. In some individuals, a breathing-related sleep disorder may precipitate episodes of sleepwalking.

REM sleep behavior disorder.   REM sleep behavior disorder may be difficult to distinguish from NREM sleep arousal disorders. REM sleep behavior disorder is characterized by episodes of prominent, complex movements, often involving personal injury arising from sleep. In contrast to NREM sleep arousal disorders, REM sleep behavior disorder occurs during REM sleep. Individuals with REM sleep behavior disorder awaken easily and report more detailed and vivid dream content than do individuals with NREM sleep arousal disorders. They often report that they "act out dreams."

Parasomnia overlap syndrome.   Parasomnia overlap syndrome consists of clinical and polysomnographic features of both sleepwalking and REM sleep behavior disorder.

Sleep-related seizures.   Some types of seizures can produce episodes of very unusual behaviors that occur predominantly or exclusively during sleep. Nocturnal seizures may closely mimic NREM sleep arousal disorders but tend to be more stereotypic in nature, occur multiple times nightly, and be more likely to occur from daytime naps. The presence of sleep-related seizures does not preclude the presence of NREM sleep arousal disorders. Sleep-related seizures should be classified as a form of epilepsy.

Alcohol-induced blackouts.   Alcohol-induced blackouts may be associated with extremely complex behaviors in the absence of other suggestions of intoxication. They do not involve the loss of consciousness but rather reflect an isolated disruption of memory for events during a drinking episode. By history, these behaviors may be indistinguishable from those seen in NREM sleep arousal disorders.

Dissociative amnesia, with dissociative fugue.   Dissociative fugue may be extremely difficult to distinguish from sleepwalking. Unlike all other parasomnias, nocturnal dissociative fugue arises from a period of wakefulness during sleep, rather than precipitously from sleep without intervening wakefulness. A history of recurrent childhood physical or sexual abuse is usually present (but may be difficult to obtain).

Malingering or other voluntary behavior occurring during wakefulness.   As with dissociative fugue, malingering or other voluntary behavior occurring during wakefulness arises from wakefulness.

Panic disorder.   Panic attacks may also cause abrupt awakenings from deep NREM sleep accompanied by fearfulness, but these episodes produce rapid and complete awakening without the confusion, amnesia, or motor activity typical of NREM sleep arousal disorders.

Medication-induced complex behaviors.   Behaviors similar to those in NREM sleep arousal disorders can be induced by use of, or withdrawal from, substances or medications (e.g., benzodiazepines, nonbenzodiazepine sedative-hypnotics, opiates, cocaine, nicotine, antipsychotics, tricyclic antidepressants, chloral hydrate). Such behaviors may arise from the sleep period and may be extremely complex. The underlying pathophysiology appears to be a relatively isolated amnesia. In such cases, substance/medication-induced sleep disorder, parasomnia type, should be diagnosed (see "Substance/Medication-Induced Sleep Disorder" later in this chapter).

Night eating syndrome.   The sleep-related eating disorder form of sleepwalking is to be differentiated from night eating syndrome, in which there is a delay in the circadian rhythm of food ingestion and an association with insomnia and/or depression.

Comorbidity

In adults, there is an association between sleepwalking and major depressive episodes and obsessive-compulsive disorder. Children or adults with sleep terrors may have elevated scores for depression and anxiety on personality inventories.

Relationship to International Classification of Sleep Disorders

The *International Classification of Sleep Disorders*, 2nd Edition, includes "confusional arousal" as a NREM sleep arousal disorder.

Nightmare Disorder

Diagnostic Criteria	307.47 (F51.5)

A. Repeated occurrences of extended, extremely dysphoric, and well-remembered dreams that usually involve efforts to avoid threats to survival, security, or physical integrity and that generally occur during the second half of the major sleep episode.
B. On awakening from the dysphoric dreams, the individual rapidly becomes oriented and alert.
C. The sleep disturbance causes clinically significant distress or impairment in social, occupational, or other important areas of functioning.
D. The nightmare symptoms are not attributable to the physiological effects of a substance (e.g., a drug of abuse, a medication).
E. Coexisting mental and medical disorders do not adequately explain the predominant complaint of dysphoric dreams.

Specify if:
  During sleep onset
Specify if:
  With associated non–sleep disorder, including substance use disorders
  With associated other medical condition
  With associated other sleep disorder
  Coding note: The code 307.47 (F51.5) applies to all three specifiers. Code also the relevant associated mental disorder, medical condition, or other sleep disorder immediately after the code for nightmare disorder in order to indicate the association.
Specify if:
  Acute: Duration of period of nightmares is 1 month or less.
  Subacute: Duration of period of nightmares is greater than 1 month but less than 6 months.
  Persistent: Duration of period of nightmares is 6 months or greater.
Specify current severity:
  Severity can be rated by the frequency with which the nightmares occur:
  Mild: Less than one episode per week on average.
  Moderate: One or more episodes per week but less than nightly.
  Severe: Episodes nightly.

Diagnostic Features

Nightmares are typically lengthy, elaborate, storylike sequences of dream imagery that seem real and that incite anxiety, fear, or other dysphoric emotions. Nightmare content typically focuses on attempts to avoid or cope with imminent danger but may involve themes that evoke other negative emotions. Nightmares occurring after traumatic experiences may replicate the threatening situation ("replicative nightmares"), but most do not. On awakening, nightmares are well remembered and can be described in detail. They arise almost exclusively during rapid eye movement (REM) sleep and can thus occur throughout sleep but are more likely in the second half of the major sleep episode when dreaming is longer and more intense. Factors that increase early-night REM intensity, such as sleep fragmentation or deprivation, jet lag, and REM-sensitive medications, might facilitate nightmares earlier in the night, including at sleep onset.

Nightmares usually terminate with awakening and rapid return of full alertness. However, the dysphoric emotions may persist into wakefulness and contribute to difficulty returning to sleep and lasting daytime distress. Some nightmares, known as "bad dreams," may not induce awakening and are recalled only later. If nightmares occur during sleep-onset REM periods (*hypnagogic*), the dysphoric emotion is frequently accompanied by a sense of being both awake and unable to move voluntarily (*isolated sleep paralysis*).

Associated Features Supporting Diagnosis

Mild autonomic arousal, including sweating, tachycardia, and tachypnea, may characterize nightmares. Body movements and vocalizations are not characteristic because of REM sleep–related loss of skeletal muscle tone, but such behaviors may occur under situations of emotional stress or sleep fragmentation and in posttraumatic stress disorder (PTSD). When talking or emoting occurs, it is typically a brief event terminating the nightmare.

Individuals with frequent nightmares are at substantially greater risk for suicidal ideation and suicide attempts, even when gender and mental illness are taken into account.

Prevalence

Prevalence of nightmares increases through childhood into adolescence. From 1.3% to 3.9% of parents report that their preschool children have nightmares "often" or "always." Prevalence increases from ages 10 to 13 for both males and females but continues to increase to ages 20–29 for females (while decreasing for males), when it can be twice as high for females as for males. Prevalence decreases steadily with age for both sexes, but the gender difference remains. Among adults, prevalence of nightmares at least monthly is 6%, whereas prevalence for frequent nightmares is 1%–2%. Estimates often combine idiopathic and posttraumatic nightmares indiscriminately.

Development and Course

Nightmares often begin between ages 3 and 6 years but reach a peak prevalence and severity in late adolescence or early adulthood. Nightmares most likely appear in children exposed to acute or chronic psychosocial stressors and thus may not resolve spontaneously. In a minority, frequent nightmares persist into adulthood, becoming virtually a lifelong disturbance. Although specific nightmare content may reflect the individual's age, the essential features of the disorder are the same across age groups.

Risk and Prognostic Factors

Temperamental. Individuals who experience nightmares report more frequent past adverse events, but not necessarily trauma, and often display personality disturbances or psychiatric diagnosis.

Environmental.   Sleep deprivation or fragmentation, and irregular sleep-wake sched-ules that alter the timing, intensity, or quantity of REM sleep, can put individuals at risk for nightmares.

Genetic and physiological.   Twin studies have identified genetic effects on the dis-position to nightmares and their co-occurrence with other parasomnias (e.g., sleep-talking).

Course modifiers.   Adaptive parental bedside behaviors, such as soothing the child following nightmares, may protect against developing chronic nightmares.

Culture-Related Diagnostic Issues

The significance attributed to nightmares may vary by culture, and sensitivity to such beliefs may facilitate disclosure.

Gender-Related Diagnostic Issues

Adult females report having nightmares more frequently than do adult males. Night-mare content differs by sex, with adult females tending to report themes of sexual harassment or of loved ones disappearing/dying, and adult males tending to report themes of physical aggression or war/terror.

Diagnostic Markers

Polysomnographic studies demonstrate abrupt awakenings from REM sleep, usually during the second half of the night, prior to report of a nightmare. Heart, respiratory, and eye movement rates may quicken or increase in variability before awakening. Night-mares following traumatic events may also arise during non-REM (NREM), particularly stage 2, sleep. The typical sleep of individuals with nightmares is mildly impaired (e.g., re-duced efficiency, less slow-wave sleep, more awakenings), with more frequent periodic leg movements in sleep and relative sympathetic nervous system activation after REM sleep deprivation.

Functional Consequences of Nightmare Disorder

Nightmares cause more significant subjective distress than demonstrable social or oc-cupational impairment. However, if awakenings are frequent or result in sleep avoid-ance, individuals may experience excessive daytime sleepiness, poor concentration, depression, anxiety, or irritability. Frequent childhood nightmares (e.g., several per week) may cause significant distress to parents and child.

Differential Diagnosis

Sleep terror disorder.   Both nightmare disorder and sleep terror disorder include awakenings or partial awakenings with fearfulness and autonomic activation, but the two disorders are differentiable. Nightmares typically occur later in the night, during REM sleep, and produce vivid, storylike, and clearly recalled dreams; mild autonomic arousal; and complete awakenings. Sleep terrors typically arise in the first third of the night during stage 3 or 4 NREM sleep and produce either no dream recall or images without an elaborate storylike quality. The terrors lead to partial awakenings that leave the individual confused, disoriented, and only partially responsive and with substantial autonomic arousal. There is usually amnesia for the event in the morning.

REM sleep behavior disorder.   The presence of complex motor activity during frightening dreams should prompt further evaluation for REM sleep behavior disorder, which occurs more typically among late middle-age males and, unlike nightmare disorder, is associated with often violent dream enactments and a history of nocturnal injuries. The dream disturbance of REM sleep behavior disorder is described by patients as nightmares but is controlled by appropriate medication.

Bereavement.   Dysphoric dreams may occur during bereavement but typically involve loss and sadness and are followed by self-reflection and insight, rather than distress, on awakening.

Narcolepsy.   Nightmares are a frequent complaint in narcolepsy, but the presence of excessive sleepiness and cataplexy differentiates this condition from nightmare disorder.

Nocturnal seizures.   Seizures may rarely manifest as nightmares and should be evaluated with polysomnography and continuous video electroencephalography. Nocturnal seizures usually involve stereotypical motor activity. Associated nightmares, if recalled, are often repetitive in nature or reflect epileptogenic features such as the content of diurnal auras (e.g., unmotivated dread), phosphenes, or ictal imagery. Disorders of arousal, especially confusional arousals, may also be present.

Breathing-related sleep disorders.   Breathing-related sleep disorders can lead to awakenings with autonomic arousal, but these are not usually accompanied by recall of nightmares.

Panic disorder.   Attacks arising during sleep can produce abrupt awakenings with autonomic arousal and fearfulness, but nightmares are typically not reported and symptoms are similar to panic attacks arising during wakefulness.

Sleep-related dissociative disorders.   Individuals may recall actual physical or emotional trauma as a "dream" during electroencephalography-documented awakenings.

Medication or substance use.   Numerous substances/medications can precipitate nightmares, including dopaminergics; beta-adrenergic antagonists and other antihypertensives; amphetamine, cocaine, and other stimulants; antidepressants; smoking cessation aids; and melatonin. Withdrawal of REM sleep–suppressant medications (e.g., antidepressants) and alcohol can produce REM sleep rebound accompanied by nightmares. If nightmares are sufficiently severe to warrant independent clinical attention, a diagnosis of substance/medication-induced sleep disorder should be considered.

Comorbidity

Nightmares may be comorbid with several medical conditions, including coronary heart disease, cancer, parkinsonism, and pain, and can accompany medical treatments, such as hemodialysis, or withdrawal from medications or substances of abuse. Nightmares frequently are comorbid with other mental disorders, including PTSD; insomnia disorder; schizophrenia; psychosis; mood, anxiety, adjustment, and personality disorders; and grief during bereavement. A concurrent nightmare disorder diagnosis should only be considered when independent clinical attention is warranted (i.e., Criteria A–C are met). Otherwise, no separate diagnosis is necessary. These conditions should be listed under the appropriate comorbid category specifier. However, nightmare disorder may be diagnosed as a separate disorder in individuals with PTSD if the nightmares are temporally unrelated to PTSD (i.e., preceding other PTSD symptoms or persisting after other PTSD symptoms have resolved).

Nightmares are normally characteristic of REM sleep behavior disorder, PTSD, and acute stress disorder, but nightmare disorder may be independently coded if nightmares preceded the condition and their frequency or severity necessitates independent clinical attention. The latter may be determined by asking whether nightmares were a problem before onset of the other disorder and whether they continued after other symptoms had remitted.

Relationship to International Classification of Sleep Disorders

The *International Classification of Sleep Disorders,* 2nd Edition (ICSD-2), presents similar diagnostic criteria for nightmare disorder.

Rapid Eye Movement Sleep Behavior Disorder

Diagnostic Criteria   **327.42 (G47.52)**

A. Repeated episodes of arousal during sleep associated with vocalization and/or complex motor behaviors.
B. These behaviors arise during rapid eye movement (REM) sleep and therefore usually occur more than 90 minutes after sleep onset, are more frequent during the later portions of the sleep period, and uncommonly occur during daytime naps.
C. Upon awakening from these episodes, the individual is completely awake, alert, and not confused or disoriented.
D. Either of the following:
    1. REM sleep without atonia on polysomnographic recording.
    2. A history suggestive of REM sleep behavior disorder and an established synucleinopathy diagnosis (e.g., Parkinson's disease, multiple system atrophy).
E. The behaviors cause clinically significant distress or impairment in social, occupational, or other important areas of functioning (which may include injury to self or the bed partner).
F. The disturbance is not attributable to the physiological effects of a substance (e.g., a drug of abuse, a medication) or another medical condition.
G. Coexisting mental and medical disorders do not explain the episodes.

Diagnostic Features

The essential feature of rapid eye movement (REM) sleep behavior disorder is repeated episodes of arousal, often associated with vocalizations and/or complex motor behaviors arising from REM sleep (Criterion A). These behaviors often reflect motor responses to the content of action-filled or violent dreams of being attacked or trying to escape from a threatening situation, which may be termed *dream enacting behaviors.* The vocalizations are often loud, emotion-filled, and profane. These behaviors may be very bothersome to the individual and the bed partner and may result in significant injury (e.g., falling, jumping, or flying out of bed; running, punching, thrusting, hitting, or kicking). Upon awakening, the individual is immediately awake, alert, and oriented (Criterion C) and is often able to recall dream mentation, which closely correlates with the observed behavior. The eyes typically remain closed during these events. The diagnosis of REM sleep behavior disorder requires clinically significant distress or impairment (Criterion E); this determination will depend on a number of factors, including the frequency of events, the potential for violence or injurious behaviors, embarrassment, and distress in other household members.

Associated Features Supporting Diagnosis

Severity determination is best made based on the nature or consequence of the behavior rather than simply on frequency. Although the behaviors are typically prominent and violent, lesser behaviors may also occur.

Prevalence

The prevalence of REM sleep behavior disorder is approximately 0.38%–0.5% in the general population. Prevalence in patients with psychiatric disorders may be greater, possibly related to medications prescribed for the psychiatric disorder.

Development and Course

The onset of REM sleep behavior disorder may be gradual or rapid, and the course is usually progressive. REM sleep behavior disorder associated with neurodegenerative disorders may improve as the underlying neurodegenerative disorder progresses. Because of the very high association with the later appearance of an underlying neurodegenerative disorder, most notably one of the synucleinopathies (Parkinson's disease, multiple system atrophy, or major or mild neurocognitive disorder with Lewy bodies), the neurological status of individuals with REM sleep behavior disorder should be closely monitored.

REM sleep behavior disorder overwhelmingly affects males older than 50 years, but increasingly this disorder is being identified in females and in younger individuals. Symptoms in young individuals, particularly young females, should raise the possibility of narcolepsy or medication-induced REM sleep behavior disorder.

Risk and Prognostic Factors

Genetic and physiological.   Many widely prescribed medications, including tricyclic antidepressants, selective serotonin reuptake inhibitors, serotonin-norepinephrine reuptake inhibitors, and beta-blockers, may result in polysomnographic evidence of REM sleep without atonia and in frank REM sleep behavior disorder. It is not known whether the medications per se result in REM sleep behavior disorder or they unmask an underlying predisposition.

Diagnostic Markers

Associated laboratory findings from polysomnography indicate increased tonic and/ or phasic electromyographic activity during REM sleep that is normally associated with muscle atonia. The increased muscle activity variably affects different muscle groups, mandating more extensive electromyographic monitoring than is employed in conventional sleep studies. For this reason, it is suggested that electromyographic monitoring include the submentalis, bilateral extensor digitorum, and bilateral anterior tibialis muscle groups. Continuous video monitoring is mandatory. Other polysomnographic findings may include very frequent periodic and aperiodic extremity electromyography activity during non-REM (NREM) sleep. This polysomnography observation, termed *REM sleep without atonia*, is present in virtually all cases of REM sleep behavior disorder but may also be an asymptomatic polysomnographic finding. Clinical dream-enacting behaviors coupled with the polysomnographic finding of REM without atonia is necessary for the diagnosis of REM sleep behavior disorder. REM sleep without atonia without a clinical history of dream-enacting behaviors is simply an asymptomatic polysomnographic observation. It is not known whether isolated REM sleep without atonia is a precursor to REM sleep behavior disorder.

Functional Consequences of Rapid Eye Movement Sleep Behavior Disorder

REM sleep behavior disorder may occur in isolated occasions in otherwise unaffected individuals. Embarrassment concerning the episodes can impair social relationships. Individuals may avoid situations in which others might become aware of the disturbance, visiting friends overnight, or sleeping with bed partners. Social isolation or occupational difficulties can result. Uncommonly, REM sleep behavior disorder may result in serious injury to the victim or to the bed partner.

Differential Diagnosis

Other parasomnias.   Confusional arousals, sleepwalking, and sleep terrors can easily be confused with REM sleep behavior disorder. In general, these disorders occur in younger individuals. Unlike REM sleep behavior disorder, they arise from deep NREM sleep and therefore tend to occur in the early portion of the sleep period. Awakening from a confusional arousal is associated with confusion, disorientation, and incomplete recall of dream mentation accompanying the behavior. Polysomnographic monitoring in the disorders of arousal reveals normal REM atonia.

Nocturnal seizures.   Nocturnal seizures may perfectly mimic REM sleep behavior disorder, but the behaviors are generally more stereotyped. Polysomnographic monitoring employing a full electroencephalographic seizure montage may differentiate the two. REM sleep without atonia is not present on polysomnographic monitoring.

Obstructive sleep apnea.   Obstructive sleep apnea may result in behaviors indistinguishable from REM sleep behavior disorder. Polysomnographic monitoring is necessary to differentiate between the two. In this case, the symptoms resolve following effective treatment of the obstructive sleep apnea, and REM sleep without atonia is not present on polysomnography monitoring.

Other specified dissociative disorder (sleep-related psychogenic dissociative disorder). Unlike virtually all other parasomnias, which arise precipitously from NREM or REM sleep, psychogenic dissociative behaviors arise from a period of well-defined wakefulness during the sleep period. Unlike REM sleep behavior disorder, this condition is more prevalent in young females.

Malingering. Many cases of malingering in which the individual reports problematic sleep movements perfectly mimic the clinical features of REM sleep behavior disorder, and polysomnographic documentation is mandatory.

Comorbidity

REM sleep behavior disorder is present concurrently in approximately 30% of patients with narcolepsy. When it occurs in narcolepsy, the demographics reflect the younger age range of narcolepsy, with equal frequency in males and females. Based on findings from individuals presenting to sleep clinics, most individuals (>50%) with initially "idiopathic" REM sleep behavior disorder will eventually develop a neurodegenerative disease—most notably, one of the synucleinopathies (Parkinson's disease, multiple system atrophy, or major or mild neurocognitive disorder with Lewy bodies). REM sleep behavior disorder often predates any other sign of these disorders by many years (often more than a decade).

Relationship to International Classification of Sleep Disorders

REM sleep behavior disorder is virtually identical to REM sleep behavior disorder in the *International Classification of Sleep Disorders,* 2nd Edition (ICSD-2).

Restless Legs Syndrome

Diagnostic Criteria **333.94 (G25.81)**

A. An urge to move the legs, usually accompanied by or in response to uncomfortable and unpleasant sensations in the legs, characterized by all of the following:

1. The urge to move the legs begins or worsens during periods of rest or inactivity.
2. The urge to move the legs is partially or totally relieved by movement.
3. The urge to move the legs is worse in the evening or at night than during the day, or occurs only in the evening or at night.

B. The symptoms in Criterion A occur at least three times per week and have persisted for at least 3 months.

C. The symptoms in Criterion A are accompanied by significant distress or impairment in social, occupational, educational, academic, behavioral, or other important areas of functioning.

D. The symptoms in Criterion A are not attributable to another mental disorder or medical condition (e.g., arthritis, leg edema, peripheral ischemia, leg cramps) and are not better explained by a behavioral condition (e.g., positional discomfort, habitual foot tapping).

E. The symptoms are not attributable to the physiological effects of a drug of abuse or medication (e.g., akathisia).

Diagnostic Features

Restless legs syndrome (RLS) is a sensorimotor, neurological sleep disorder characterized by a desire to move the legs or arms, usually associated with uncomfortable
sensations typically described as creeping, crawling, tingling, burning, or itching (Criterion A). The diagnosis of RLS is based primarily on patient self-report and history.
Symptoms are worse when the individual is at rest, and frequent movements of the legs
occur in an effort to relieve the uncomfortable sensations. Symptoms are worse in the
evening or night, and in some individuals they occur only in the evening or night. Evening worsening occurs independently of any differences in activity. It is important to
differentiate RLS from other conditions such as positional discomfort and leg cramps
(Criterion D).

The symptoms of RLS can delay sleep onset and awaken the individual from sleep
and are associated with significant sleep fragmentation. The relief obtained from mov-
ing the legs may no longer be apparent in severe cases. RLS is associated with daytime
sleepiness and is frequently accompanied by significant clinical distress or functional
impairment.

Associated Features Supporting Diagnosis

Periodic leg movements in sleep (PLMS) can serve as corroborating evidence for RLS,
with up to 90% of individuals diagnosed with RLS demonstrating PLMS when record-
ings are taken over multiple nights. Periodic leg movements during wakefulness are
supportive of an RLS diagnosis. Reports of difficulty initiating and maintaining sleep
and of excessive daytime sleepiness may also support the diagnosis of RLS. Additional
supportive features include a family history of RLS among first-degree relatives and a
reduction in symptoms, at least initially, with dopaminergic treatment.

Prevalence

Prevalence rates of RLS vary widely when broad criteria are utilized but range from
2% to 7.2% when more defined criteria are employed. When frequency of symptoms
is at least three times per week with moderate or severe distress, the prevalence rate is
1.6%; when frequency of symptoms is a minimum of one time per week, the prevalence
rate is 4.5%. Females are 1.5–2 times more likely than males to have RLS. RLS also increases with age. The prevalence of RLS may be lower in Asian populations.

Development and Course

The onset of RLS typically occurs in the second or third decade. Approximately 40%
of individuals diagnosed with RLS during adulthood report having experienced
symptoms before age 20 years, and 20% report having experienced symptoms before
age 10 years. Prevalence rates of RLS increase steadily with age until about age 60 years,
with symptoms remaining stable or decreasing slightly in older age groups. Compared
with nonfamilial cases, familial RLS usually has a younger age at onset and a slower
progressive course. The clinical course of RLS differs by age at onset. When onset occurs before age 45, there is often a slow progression of symptoms. In late-onset RLS,

rapid progression is typical, and aggravating factors are common. Symptoms of RLS appear similar across the lifespan, remaining stable or decreasing slightly in older age groups.

Diagnosis of RLS in children can be difficult because of the self-report component. While Criterion A for adults assumes that the description of "urge to move" is by the patient, pediatric diagnosis requires a description in the child's own words rather than by a parent or caretaker. Typically children age 6 years or older are able to provide detailed, adequate descriptors of RLS. However, children rarely use or understand the word "urge," reporting instead that their legs "have to" or "got to" move. Also, potentially related to prolonged periods of sitting during class, two-thirds of children and adolescents report daytime leg sensations. Thus, for diagnostic Criterion A3, it is important to compare equal duration of sitting or lying down in the day to sitting or lying down in the evening or night. Nocturnal worsening tends to persist even in the context of pediatric RLS. As with RLS in adults, there is a significant negative impact on sleep, mood, cognition, and function. Impairment in children and adolescents is manifested more often in behavioral and educational domains.

Risk and Prognostic Factors

Genetic and physiological.   Predisposing factors include female gender, advancing age, genetic risk variants, and family history of RLS. Precipitating factors are often time-limited, such as iron deficiency, with most individuals resuming normal sleep patterns after the initial triggering event has disappeared. Genetic risk variants also play a role in RLS secondary to such disorders as uremia, suggesting that individuals with a genetic susceptibility develop RLS in the presence of further risk factors. RLS has a strong familial component.

There are defined pathophysiological pathways subserving RLS. Genome-wide association studies have found that RLS is significantly associated with common genetic variants in intronic or intergenic regions in *MEIS1*, *BTBD9*, and *MAP2K5* on chromosomes 2p, 6p, and 15q, respectively. The association of these three variants with RLS has been independently replicated. *BTBD9* confers a very large (80%) excessive risk when even a single allele is present. Because of the high frequency of this variant in individuals of European descent, the population attributable risk (PAR) approximates 50%. At-risk alleles associated with *MEIS1* and *BTBD9* are less common in individuals of African or Asian descent, perhaps suggesting lower risk for RLS in these populations.

Pathophysiological mechanisms in RLS also include disturbances in the central dopaminergic system and disturbances in iron metabolism. The endogenous opiate system may also be involved. Treatment effects of dopaminergic drugs (primarily D_2 and D_3 non-ergot agonists) provide further support that RLS is grounded in dysfunctional central dopaminergic pathways. While the effective treatment of RLS has also been shown to significantly reduce depressive symptoms, serotonergic antidepressants can induce or aggravate RLS in some individuals.

Gender-Related Diagnostic Issues

Although RLS is more prevalent in females than in males, there are no diagnostic differences according to gender. However, the prevalence of RLS during pregnancy is two to three times greater than in the general population. RLS associated with pregnancy peaks during the third trimester and improves or resolves in most cases soon after delivery. The gender difference in prevalence of RLS is explained at least in part by parity, with nulliparous females being at the same risk of RLS as age-matched males.

Diagnostic Markers

Polysomnography demonstrates significant abnormalities in RLS, commonly increased latency to sleep, and higher arousal index. Polysomnography with a preceding immobilization test may provide an indicator of the motor sign of RLS, periodic limb movements, under standard conditions of sleep and during quiet resting, both of which can provoke RLS symptoms.

Functional Consequences of Restless Legs Syndrome

Forms of RLS severe enough to significantly impair functioning or associated with mental disorders, including depression and anxiety, occur in approximately 2%–3% of the population.

Although the impact of milder symptoms is less well characterized, individuals with RLS complain of disruption in at least one activity of daily living, with up to 50% reporting a negative impact on mood, and 47.6% reporting a lack of energy. The most common consequences of RLS are sleep disturbance, including reduced sleep time, sleep fragmentation, and overall disturbance; depression, generalized anxiety disorder, panic disorder, and posttraumatic stress disorder; and quality-of-life impairments. RLS can result in daytime sleepiness or fatigue and is frequently accompanied by significant distress or impairment in affective, social, occupational, educational, academic, behavioral, or cognitive functioning.

Differential Diagnosis

The most important conditions in the differential diagnosis of RLS are leg cramps, positional discomfort, arthralgias/arthritis, myalgias, positional ischemia (numbness), leg edema, peripheral neuropathy, radiculopathy, and habitual foot tapping. "Knotting" of the muscle (cramps), relief with a single postural shift, limitation to joints, soreness to palpation (myalgias), and other abnormalities on physical examination are not characteristic of RLS. Unlike RLS, nocturnal leg cramps do not typically present with the desire to move the limbs nor are there frequent limb movements. Less common conditions to be differentiated from RLS include neuroleptic-induced akathisia, myelopathy, symptomatic venous insufficiency, peripheral artery disease, eczema, other orthopedic problems, and anxiety-induced restlessness. Worsening at night and periodic limb movements are more common in RLS than in medication-induced akathisia or peripheral neuropathy.

While is it important that RLS symptoms not be solely accounted for by another medical or behavioral condition, it should also be appreciated that any of these similar conditions can occur in an individual with RLS. This necessitates a separate focus on each possible condition in the diagnostic process and when assessing impact. For cases in which the diagnosis of RLS is not certain, evaluation for the supportive features of RLS, particularly PLMS or a family history of RLS, may be helpful. Clinical features, such as response to a dopaminergic agent and positive family history for RLS, can help with the differential diagnosis.

Comorbidity

Depressive disorders, anxiety disorders, and attentional disorders are commonly co-morbid with RLS and are discussed in the section "Functional Consequences of Restless Legs Syndrome." The main medical disorder comorbid with RLS is cardiovascular disease. There may be an association with numerous other medical disorders, including hypertension, narcolepsy, migraine, Parkinson's disease, multiple sclerosis, peripheral neuropathy, obstructive sleep apnea, diabetes mellitus, fibromyalgia, osteoporosis, obesity, thyroid disease, and cancer. Iron deficiency, pregnancy, and chronic renal failure are also comorbid with RLS.

Relationship to International Classification of Sleep Disorders

The *International Classification of Sleep Disorders,* 2nd Edition (ICSD-2), presents similar diagnostic criteria for RLS but does not contain a criterion specifying frequency or duration of symptoms.

Substance/Medication-Induced Sleep Disorder

Diagnostic Criteria

A. A prominent and severe disturbance in sleep.

B. There is evidence from the history, physical examination, or laboratory findings of both (1) and (2):

1. The symptoms in Criterion A developed during or soon after substance intoxication or after withdrawal from or exposure to a medication.

2. The involved substance/medication is capable of producing the symptoms in Criterion A.

C. The disturbance is not better explained by a sleep disorder that is not substance/medication-induced. Such evidence of an independent sleep disorder could include the following:

The symptoms precede the onset of the substance/medication use; the symptoms persist for a substantial period of time (e.g., about 1 month) after the cessation of acute withdrawal or severe intoxication; or there is other evidence suggesting the existence of an independent non-substance/medication-induced sleep disorder (e.g., a history of recurrent non-substance/medication-related episodes).

D. The disturbance does not occur exclusively during the course of a delirium.

E. The disturbance causes clinically significant distress or impairment in social, occupational, or other important areas of functioning.

Note: This diagnosis should be made instead of a diagnosis of substance intoxication or substance withdrawal only when the symptoms in Criterion A predominate in the clinical picture and when they are sufficiently severe to warrant clinical attention.

Coding note: The ICD-9-CM and ICD-10-CM codes for the [specific substance/medication]-induced sleep disorders are indicated in the table below. Note that the ICD-10-CM code depends on whether or not there is a comorbid substance use disorder present for the same class of substance. If a mild substance use disorder is comorbid with the substance-induced sleep disorder, the 4th position character is "1," and the clinician should record "mild [substance] use disorder" before the substance-induced sleep disorder (e.g., "mild cocaine use disorder with cocaine-induced sleep disorder"). If a moderate or severe substance use disorder is comorbid with the substance-induced sleep disorder, the 4th position character is "2," and the clinician should record "moderate [substance] use disorder" or "severe [substance] use disorder," depending on the severity of the comorbid substance use disorder. If there is no comorbid substance use disorder (e.g., after a one-time heavy use of the substance), then the 4th position character is "9," and the clinician should record only the substance-induced sleep disorder. A moderate or severe tobacco use disorder is required in order to code a tobacco-induced sleep disorder; it is not permissible to code a comorbid mild tobacco use disorder or no tobacco use disorder with a tobacco-induced sleep disorder.

| | | ICD-10-CM | | |
	ICD-9-CM	With use disorder, mild	With use disorder, moderate or severe	Without use disorder
Alcohol	291.82	F10.182	F10.282	F10.982
Caffeine	292.85	F15.182	F15.282	F15.982
Cannabis	292.85	F12.188	F12.288	F12.988
Opioid	292.85	F11.182	F11.282	F11.982
Sedative, hypnotic, or anxiolytic	292.85	F13.182	F13.282	F13.982
Amphetamine (or other stimulant)	292.85	F15.182	F15.282	F15.982
Cocaine	292.85	F14.182	F14.282	F14.982
Tobacco	292.85	NA	F17.208	NA
Other (or unknown) substance	292.85	F19.182	F19.282	F19.982

Specify whether:
   Insomnia type: Characterized by difficulty falling asleep or maintaining sleep, frequent nocturnal awakenings, or nonrestorative sleep.
   Daytime sleepiness type: Characterized by predominant complaint of excessive sleepiness/fatigue during waking hours or, less commonly, a long sleep period.

Parasomnia type: Characterized by abnormal behavioral events during sleep.

Mixed type: Characterized by a substance/medication-induced sleep problem characterized by multiple types of sleep symptoms, but no symptom clearly predominates.

Specify if (see Table 1 in the chapter "Substance-Related and Addictive Disorders" [in DSM-5] for diagnoses associated with substance class):

With onset during intoxication: This specifier should be used if criteria are met for intoxication with the substance/medication and symptoms developed during the intoxication period.

With onset during discontinuation/withdrawal: This specifier should be used if criteria are met for discontinuation/withdrawal from the substance/medication and symptoms developed during, or shortly after, discontinuation of the substance/medication.

Recording Procedures

ICD-9-CM. The name of the substance/medication-induced sleep disorder begins with the specific substance (e.g., cocaine, bupropion) that is presumed to be causing the sleep disturbance. The diagnostic code is selected from the table included in the criteria set, which is based on the drug class. For substances that do not fit into any of the classes (e.g., bupropion), the code for "other substance" should be used; and in cases in which a substance is judged to be an etiological factor but the specific class of substance is unknown, the category "unknown substance" should be used.

The name of the disorder is followed by the specification of onset (i.e., onset during intoxication, onset during discontinuation/withdrawal), followed by the subtype designation (i.e., insomnia type, daytime sleepiness type, parasomnia type, mixed type). Unlike the recording procedures for ICD-10-CM, which combine the substance-induced disorder and substance use disorder into a single code, for ICD-9-CM a separate diagnostic code is given for the substance use disorder. For example, in the case of insomnia occurring during withdrawal in a man with a severe lorazepam use disorder, the diagnosis is 292.85 lorazepam-induced sleep disorder, with onset during withdrawal, insomnia type. An additional diagnosis of 304.10 severe lorazepam use disorder is also given. When more than one substance is judged to play a significant role in the development of the sleep disturbance, each should be listed separately (e.g., 292.85 alcohol-induced sleep disorder, with onset during intoxication, insomnia type; 292.85 cocaine-induced sleep disorder, with onset during intoxication, insomnia type).

ICD-10-CM. The name of the substance/medication-induced sleep disorder begins with the specific substance (e.g., cocaine, bupropion) that is presumed to be causing the sleep disturbance. The diagnostic code is selected from the table included in the criteria set, which is based on the drug class and presence or absence of a comorbid substance use disorder. For substances that do not fit into any of the classes (e.g., bupropion), the code for "other substance" should be used; and in cases in which a substance is judged to be an etiological factor but the specific class of substance is unknown, the category "unknown substance" should be used.

When recording the name of the disorder, the comorbid substance use disorder (if any) is listed first, followed by the word "with," followed by the name of the substance-induced sleep disorder, followed by the specification of onset (i.e., onset during intoxication, onset during discontinuation/withdrawal), followed by the subtype designation (i.e., insomnia type, daytime sleepiness type, parasomnia type, mixed type). For example, in the case of insomnia occurring during withdrawal in a man with a severe lorazepam use disorder, the diagnosis is F13.282 severe lorazepam use disorder with lorazepam-induced sleep disorder, with onset during withdrawal, insomnia type. A separate diagnosis of the comorbid severe lorazepam use disorder is not given. If the substance-induced sleep disorder occurs without a comorbid substance use disorder (e.g., with medication use), no accompanying substance use disorder is noted (e.g., F19.982 bupropion-induced sleep disorder, with onset during medication use, insomnia type). When more than one substance is judged to play a significant role in the development of the sleep disturbance, each should be listed separately (e.g., F10.282 severe alcohol use disorder with alcohol-induced sleep disorder, with onset during intoxication, insomnia type; F14.282 severe cocaine use disorder with cocaine-induced sleep disorder, with onset during intoxication, insomnia type).

Diagnostic Features

The essential feature of substance/medication-induced sleep disorder is a prominent sleep disturbance that is sufficiently severe to warrant independent clinical attention (Criterion A) and that is judged to be primarily associated with the pharmacological effects of a substance (i.e., a drug of abuse, a medication, toxin exposure) (Criterion B). Depending on the substance involved, one of four types of sleep disturbances is reported. Insomnia type and daytime sleepiness type are most common, while parasomnia type is seen less often. The mixed type is noted when more than one type of sleep disturbance–related symptom is present and none predominates. The disturbance must not be better explained by another sleep disorder (Criterion C). A substance/medication-induced sleep disorder is distinguished from insomnia disorder or a disorder associated with excessive daytime sleepiness by considering onset and course. For drugs of abuse, there must be evidence of intoxication or withdrawal from the history, physical examination, or laboratory findings. Substance/medication-induced sleep disorder arises only in association with intoxication or discontinuation/withdrawal states, whereas other sleep disorders may precede the onset of substance use or occur during times of sustained abstinence. As discontinuation/withdrawal states for some substances can be protracted, onset of the sleep disturbance can occur 4 weeks after cessation of substance use, and the disturbance may have features atypical of other sleep disorders (e.g., atypical age at onset or course). The diagnosis is not made if the sleep disturbance occurs only during a delirium (Criterion D). The symptoms must cause clinically significant distress or impairment in social, occupational, or other important areas of functioning (Criterion E). This diagnosis should be made instead of a diagnosis of substance intoxication or substance withdrawal only when the symptoms in Criterion A predominate in the clinical picture and when the symptoms warrant independent clinical attention.

Associated Features Supporting Diagnosis

During periods of substance/medication use, intoxication, or withdrawal, individuals frequently complain of dysphoric mood, including depression and anxiety, irritability, cognitive impairment, inability to concentrate, and fatigue.

Prominent and severe sleep disturbances can occur in association with intoxication with the following classes of substances: alcohol; caffeine; cannabis; opioids; sedatives, hypnotics, or anxiolytics; stimulants (including cocaine); and other (or unknown) substances. Prominent and severe sleep disturbances can occur in association with withdrawal from the following classes of substances: alcohol; caffeine; cannabis; opioids; sedatives, hypnotics, or anxiolytics; stimulant (including cocaine); tobacco; and other (or unknown) substances. Some medications that invoke sleep disturbances include adrenergic agonists and antagonists, dopamine agonists and antagonists, cholinergic agonists and antagonists, serotonergic agonists and antagonists, antihistamines, and corticosteroids.

Alcohol.   Alcohol-induced sleep disorder typically occurs as insomnia type. During acute intoxication, alcohol produces an immediate sedative effect depending on dose, accompanied by increased stages 3 and 4 non–rapid eye movement (NREM) sleep and reduced rapid eye movement (REM) sleep. Following these initial effects, there may be increased wakefulness, restless sleep, and vivid and anxiety-laden dreams for the remaining sleep period. In parallel, stages 3 and 4 sleep are reduced, and wakefulness and REM sleep are increased. Alcohol can aggravate breathing-related sleep disorder. With habitual use, alcohol continues to show a short-lived sedative effect in the first half of the night, followed by sleep continuity disruption in the second half. During alcohol withdrawal, there is extremely disrupted sleep continuity, and an increased amount and intensity of REM sleep, associated frequently with vivid dreaming, which in extreme form, constitutes part of alcohol withdrawal delirium. After acute withdrawal, chronic alcohol users may continue to complain of light, fragmented sleep for weeks to years associated with a persistent deficit in slow-wave sleep.

Caffeine.   Caffeine-induced sleep disorder produces insomnia in a dose-dependent manner, with some individuals presenting with daytime sleepiness related to withdrawal.

Cannabis.   Acute administration of cannabis may shorten sleep latency, though arousing effects with increments in sleep latency also occur. Cannabis enhances slow-wave sleep and suppresses REM sleep after acute administration. In chronic users, tolerance to the sleep-inducing and slow-wave sleep–enhancing effects develops. Upon withdrawal, sleep difficulties and unpleasant dreams have been reported lasting for several weeks. Polysomnography studies demonstrate reduced slow-wave sleep and increased REM sleep during this phase.

Opioids.   Opioids may produce an increase in sleepiness and in subjective depth of sleep, and reduced REM sleep, during acute short-term use. With continued administration, tolerance to the sedative effects of opioids develops and there are complaints of insomnia. Consistent with their respiratory depressant effects, opioids exacerbate sleep apnea.

Sedative, hypnotic, or anxiolytic substances.   Sedatives, hypnotics, and anxiolytics (e.g., barbiturates, benzodiazepines receptor agonists, meprobamate, glutethimide, methyprylon) have similar effects as opioids on sleep. During acute intoxication, sedative-hypnotic drugs produce the expected increase in sleepiness and decrease in wakefulness. Chronic use (particularly of barbiturates and the older nonbarbiturate, nonbenzodiazepine drugs) may cause tolerance with subsequent return of insomnia. Daytime sleepiness may occur. Sedative-hypnotic drugs can increase the frequency and severity of obstructive sleep apnea events. Parasomnias are associated with use of benzodiazepine receptor agonists, especially when these medications are taken at higher doses and when they are combined with other sedative drugs. Abrupt discontinuation of chronic sedative, hypnotic, or anxiolytic use can lead to withdrawal but more commonly rebound insomnia, a condition of an exacerbation of insomnia upon drug discontinuation for 1–2 days reported to occur even with short-term use. Sedative, hypnotic, or anxiolytic drugs with short durations of action are most likely to produce complaints of rebound insomnia, whereas those with longer durations of action are more often associated with daytime sleepiness. Any sedative, hypnotic, or anxiolytic drug can potentially cause daytime sedation, withdrawal, or rebound insomnia.

Amphetamines and related substances and other stimulants.   Sleep disorders induced by amphetamine and related substances and other stimulants are characterized by insomnia during intoxication and excessive sleepiness during withdrawal. During acute intoxication, stimulants reduce the total amount of sleep, increase sleep latency and sleep continuity disturbances, and decrease REM sleep. Slow-wave sleep tends to be reduced. During withdrawal from chronic stimulant use, there is both prolonged nocturnal sleep duration and excessive daytime sleepiness. Multiple sleep latency tests may show increased daytime sleepiness during the withdrawal phase. Drugs like 3,4-methylenedioxymethamphetamine (MDMA; "ecstasy") and related substances lead to restless and disturbed sleep within 48 hours of intake; frequent use of these compounds is associated with persisting symptoms of anxiety, depression, and sleep disturbances, even during longer-term abstinence.

Tobacco.   Chronic tobacco consumption is associated primarily with symptoms of insomnia, decreased slow-wave sleep with a reduction of sleep efficiency, and increased daytime sleepiness. Withdrawal from tobacco can lead to impaired sleep. Individuals who smoke heavily may experience regular nocturnal awakenings caused by tobacco craving.

Other or unknown substances/medications.   Other substances/medications may produce sleep disturbances, particularly medications that affect the central or autonomic nervous systems (e.g., adrenergic agonists and antagonists, dopamine agonists and antagonists, cholinergic agonists and antagonists, serotonergic agonists and antagonists, antihistamines, corticosteroids).

Development and Course

Insomnia in children can be identified by either a parent or the child. Often the child has a clear sleep disturbance associated with initiation of a medication but may not report symptoms, although parents observe the sleep disturbances. The use of some illicit substances (e.g., cannabis, ecstasy) is prevalent in adolescence and early adulthood. Insomnia or any other sleep disturbance encountered in this age group should prompt careful consideration of whether the sleep disturbance is due to consumption of these substances. Help-seeking behavior for the sleep disturbance in these age groups is limited, and thus corroborative report may be elicited from a parent, caregiver, or teacher. Older individuals take more medications and are at increased risk for developing a substance/medication-induced sleep disorder. They may interpret sleep disturbance as part of normal aging and fail to report symptoms. Individuals with major neurocognitive disorder (e.g., dementia) are at risk for substance/medication-induced sleep disorders but may not report symptoms, making corroborative report from caregiver(s) particularly important.

Risk and Prognostic Factors

Risk and prognostic factors involved in substance abuse/dependence or medication use are normative for certain age groups. They are relevant for, and likely applicable to, the type of sleep disturbance encountered (see the chapter "Substance-Related and Addictive Disorders" [in DSM-5] for descriptions of respective substance use disorders).

Temperamental.   Substance use generally precipitates or accompanies insomnia in vulnerable individuals. Thus, presence of insomnia in response to stress or change in sleep environment or timing can represent a risk for developing substance/medication-induced sleep disorder. A similar risk may be present for individuals with other sleep disorders (e.g., individuals with hypersomnia who use stimulants).

Culture-Related Diagnostic Issues

The consumption of substances, including prescribed medications, may depend in part on cultural background and specific local drug regulations.

Gender-Related Diagnostic Issues

Gender-specific prevalences (i.e., females affected more than males at a ratio of about 2:1) exist for patterns of consumption of some substances (e.g., alcohol). The same amount and duration of consumption of a given substance may lead to highly different sleep-related outcomes in males and females based on, for example, gender-specific differences in hepatic functioning.

Diagnostic Markers

Each of the substance/medication-induced sleep disorders produces electroencephalographic sleep patterns that are associated with, but cannot be considered diagnostic of, other disorders. The electroencephalographic sleep profile for each substance is related to the stage of use, whether intake/intoxication, chronic use, or withdrawal following discontinuation of the substance. All-night polysomnography can help define the severity of insomnia complaints, while the multiple sleep latency test provides information about the severity of daytime sleepiness. Monitoring of nocturnal respiration and periodic limb movements with polysomnography may verify a substance's impact on nocturnal breathing and motor behavior. Sleep diaries for 2 weeks and actigraphy are considered helpful in confirming the presence of substance/medication-induced sleep disorder. Drug screening can be of use when the individual is not aware or unwilling to relate information about substance intake.

Functional Consequences of Substance/Medication-Induced Sleep Disorder

While there are many functional consequences associated with sleep disorders, the only unique consequence for substance/medication-induced sleep disorder is increased risk for relapse. The degree of sleep disturbance during alcohol withdrawal (e.g., REM sleep rebound predicts risk of relapse of drinking). Monitoring of sleep quality and daytime sleepiness during and after withdrawal may provide clinically meaningful information on whether an individual is at increased risk for relapse.

Differential Diagnosis

Substance intoxication or substance withdrawal.   Sleep disturbances are commonly encountered in the context of substance intoxication or substance discontinuation/withdrawal. A diagnosis of substance/medication-induced sleep disorder should be made instead of a diagnosis of substance intoxication or substance withdrawal only when the sleep disturbance is predominant in the clinical picture and is sufficiently severe to warrant independent clinical attention.

Delirium.   If the substance/medication-induced sleep disturbance occurs exclusively during the course of a delirium, it is not diagnosed separately.

Other sleep disorders.   A substance/medication-induced sleep disorder is distinguished from another sleep disorder if a substance/medication is judged to be etiologically related to the symptoms. A substance/medication-induced sleep disorder attributed to a prescribed medication for a mental disorder or medical condition must have its onset while the individual is receiving the medication or during discontinuation, if there is a discontinuation/withdrawal syndrome associated with the medication. Once treatment is discontinued, the sleep disturbance will usually remit within days to several weeks. If symptoms persist beyond 4 weeks, other causes for the sleep disturbance–related symptoms should be considered. Not infrequently, individuals with another sleep disorder use medications or drugs of abuse to self-medicate their symptoms (e.g., alcohol for management of insomnia). If the substance/medication is judged to play a significant role in the exacerbation of the sleep disturbance, an additional diagnosis of a substance/medication-induced sleep disorder may be warranted.

Sleep disorder due to another medical condition.   Substance/medication-induced sleep disorder and sleep disorder associated with another medical condition may produce similar symptoms of insomnia, daytime sleepiness, or a parasomnia. Many individuals with other medical conditions that cause sleep disturbance are treated with medications that may also cause sleep disturbances. The chronology of symptoms is the most important factor in distinguishing between these two sources of sleep symptoms. Difficulties with sleep that clearly preceded the use of any medication for treatment of a medical condition would suggest a diagnosis of sleep disorder associated with another medical condition. Conversely, sleep symptoms that appear only after the initiation of a particular medication/substance suggest a substance/medication-induced sleep disorder. If the disturbance is comorbid with another medical condition and is also exacerbated by substance use, both diagnoses (i.e., sleep disorder associated with another medical condition and substance/medication-induced sleep disorder) are given. When there is insufficient evidence to determine whether the sleep disturbance is attributable to a substance/medication or to another medical condition or is primary (i.e., not due to either a substance/medication or another medical condition), a diagnosis of other specified sleep-wake disorder or unspecified sleep-wake disorder is indicated.

Comorbidity

See the "Comorbidity" sections for other sleep disorders in this chapter, including insomnia, hypersomnolence, central sleep apnea, sleep-related hypoventilation, and circadian rhythm sleep-wake disorders, shift work type.

Relationship to International Classification of Sleep Disorders

The *International Classification of Sleep Disorders*, 2nd Edition (ICSD-2), lists sleep disorders "due to drug or substance" under their respective phenotypes (e.g., insomnia, hypersomnia).

Other Specified Insomnia Disorder

780.52 (G47.09)

This category applies to presentations in which symptoms characteristic of insomnia disorder that cause clinically significant distress or impairment in social, occupational, or other important areas of functioning predominate but do not meet the full criteria for insomnia disorder or any of the disorders in the sleep-wake disorders diagnostic class. The other specified insomnia disorder category is used in situations in which the clinician chooses to communicate the specific reason that the presentation does not meet the criteria for insomnia disorder or any specific sleep-wake disorder. This is done by recording "other specified insomnia disorder" followed by the specific reason (e.g., "brief insomnia disorder").

Examples of presentations that can be specified using the "other specified" designation include the following:

1. **Brief insomnia disorder:** Duration is less than 3 months.
2. **Restricted to nonrestorative sleep:** Predominant complaint is nonrestorative sleep unaccompanied by other sleep symptoms such as difficulty falling asleep or remaining asleep.

Unspecified Insomnia Disorder

780.52 (G47.00)

This category applies to presentations in which symptoms characteristic of insomnia disorder that cause clinically significant distress or impairment in social, occupational, or other important areas of functioning predominate but do not meet the full criteria for insomnia disorder or any of the disorders in the sleep-wake disorders diagnostic class. The unspecified insomnia disorder category is used in situations in which the clinician chooses *not* to specify the reason that the criteria are not met for insomnia disorder or a specific sleep-wake disorder, and includes presentations in which there is insufficient information to make a more specific diagnosis.

Other Specified Hypersomnolence Disorder

780.54 (G47.19)

This category applies to presentations in which symptoms characteristic of hypersomnolence disorder that cause clinically significant distress or impairment in social, occupational, or other important areas of functioning predominate but do not meet the full criteria for hypersomnolence disorder or any of the disorders in the sleep-wake disorders diagnostic class. The other specified hypersomnolence disorder category is used in situations in which the clinician chooses to communicate the specific reason that the presentation does not meet the criteria for hypersomnolence disorder or any specific sleep-wake disorder. This is done by recording "other specified hypersomnolence disorder" followed by the specific reason (e.g., "brief-duration hypersomnolence," as in Kleine-Levin syndrome).

Unspecified Hypersomnolence Disorder

780.54 (G47.10)

This category applies to presentations in which symptoms characteristic of hypersomnolence disorder that cause clinically significant distress or impairment in social, occupational, or other important areas of functioning predominate but do not meet the full criteria for hypersomnolence disorder or any of the disorders in the sleep-wake disorders diagnostic class. The unspecified hypersomnolence disorder category is used in situations in which the clinician chooses *not* to specify the reason that the criteria are not met for hypersomnolence disorder or a specific sleep-wake disorder, and includes presentations in which there is insufficient information to make a more specific diagnosis.

Other Specified Sleep-Wake Disorder

780.59 (G47.8)

This category applies to presentations in which symptoms characteristic of a sleep-wake disorder that cause clinically significant distress or impairment in social, occupational, or other important areas of functioning predominate but do not meet the full criteria for any of the disorders in the sleep-wake disorders diagnostic class and do not qualify for a diagnosis of other specified insomnia disorder or other specified hypersomnolence disorder. The other specified sleep-wake disorder category is used in situations in which the clinician chooses to communicate the specific reason that the presentation does not meet the criteria for any specific sleep-wake disorder. This is done by recording "other specified sleep-wake disorder" followed by the specific reason (e.g., "repeated arousals during rapid eye movement sleep without polysomnography or history of Parkinson's disease or other synucleinopathy").

Unspecified Sleep-Wake Disorder

780.59 (G47.9)

This category applies to presentations in which symptoms characteristic of a sleep-wake disorder that cause clinically significant distress or impairment in social, occupational, or other important areas of functioning predominate but do not meet the full criteria for any of the disorders in the sleep-wake disorders diagnostic class and do not qualify for a diagnosis of unspecified insomnia disorder or unspecified hypersomnolence disorder. The unspecified sleep-wake disorder category is used in situations in which the clinician chooses *not* to specify the reason that the criteria are not met for a specific sleep-wake disorder, and includes presentations in which there is insufficient information to make a more specific diagnosis.

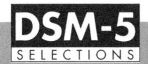

Sleep-Wake Disorders
DSM-5® Guidebook

307.42 (F51.01) Insomnia Disorder
307.44 (F51.11) Hypersomnolence Disorder
Narcolepsy

Breathing-Related Sleep Disorders
327.23 (G47.33) Obstructive Sleep Apnea Hypopnea
Central Sleep Apnea
327.2_ (G47.3_) Sleep-Related Hypoventilation

Circadian Rhythm Sleep-Wake Disorders
307.45 (G47.21) Delayed Sleep Phase Type
307.45 (G47.22) Advanced Sleep Phase Type
307.45 (G47.23) Irregular Sleep-Wake Type
307.45 (G47.24) Non-24-Hour Sleep-Wake Type
307.45 (G47.26) Shift Work Type
307.45 (G47.20) Unspecified Type

Parasomnias
Non–Rapid Eye Movement Sleep Arousal Disorders
307.46 (F51.3)   Sleepwalking Type
307.46 (F51.4)   Sleep Terror Type
307.47 (F51.5) Nightmare Disorder
327.42 (G47.52) Rapid Eye Movement Sleep Behavior Disorder
333.94 (G25.81) Restless Legs Syndrome

Substance/Medication-Induced Sleep Disorder
780.52 (G47.09) Other Specified Insomnia Disorder
780.52 (G47.00) Unspecified Insomnia Disorder
780.54 (G47.19) Other Specified Hypersomnolence Disorder
780.54 (G47.10) Unspecified Hypersomnolence Disorder
780.59 (G47.8) Other Specified Sleep-Wake Disorder
780.59 (G47.9) Unspecified Sleep-Wake Disorder

Dysfunction in sleep or waking is among the most common reasons people seek health care. The maintenance of a normal cycle of sleep and wakefulness is an important component of successful adaptation across the life cycle because robust circadian rhythms help regulate mood and enhance cognitive performance. Problems with sleep, sleep quality, and daytime alertness have enormous impact on quality of life and level of functioning.

The four stages of sleep include rapid eye movement (REM) sleep and three stages of non–rapid eye movement (NREM) sleep. Stage 1 NREM sleep is characterized by the disappearance of alpha waves and the appearance of theta waves on the electroencephalogram (EEG). Hypnic jerks are common in this stage. In stage 2 NREM sleep, sleep spindles and K-complexes are found on the EEG. Previously separated into two stages, stage 3 NREM sleep is *slow-wave sleep,* or deep sleep. Delta waves are seen on the EEG. Dreaming is more common in this stage than in other stages of NREM sleep but not as common as in REM sleep. REM sleep is characterized by rapid eye movement, low muscle tone, and rapid, low-voltage electroencephalographic activity. REM sleep alternates with periods of NREM sleep approximately every 90 minutes; in adults, REM sleep typically occupies 20%–25% of total sleep. During a normal night's sleep, most adults experience four to five periods of REM sleep. The REM episodes increase in duration during the night. The relative amount of REM sleep varies with age, with older age associated with less efficient sleep and less time spent in REM sleep.

Dysfunction in any of these sleep stages may result in a sleep-wake disorder. DSM has long recognized sleep disorders in some fashion. Somnambulism, or sleepwalking disorder, was the first sleep-wake disorder included in DSM-I. The disorder name was changed to disorder of sleep in DSM-II. DSM-III included both sleepwalking disorder and sleep terror disorder, but they were placed with the "Disorders Usually First Diagnosed in Infancy, Childhood, or Adolescence." A stand-alone chapter was developed for DSM-III-R and included the variety of disorders that are now recognized as sleep disorders. Several disorders were added to DSM-IV, such as narcolepsy and breathing-related sleep disorder.

DSM-5 recognizes 12 specific sleep-wake disorders as well as several other specified and unspecified disorders (Table 1). The chapter revision has been influenced by the second edition of the *International Classification of Sleep Disorders* (ICSD-2), published by the American Academy of Sleep Medicine (2005). The ICSD-2 contains over 70 specific sleep-wake diagnoses grouped into eight categories: insomnia, breathing-related sleep disorders, hypersomnias of central origin, circadian rhythm sleep disorders, parasomnias, sleep-related movement disorders, isolated symptoms and normal variants, and other sleep disorders. Although DSM-5 has not incorporated as many diagnoses as are contained in the ICSD-2, the current diagnoses are compatible with them.

The revisions in DSM-5 present a clinically useful approach to diagnosis. In DSM-IV, sleep disorders required the clinician to determine if the sleeping problem was a primary issue or a consequence of another problem. In DSM-5, use of the term *primary* has been dropped in favor of simply listing insomnia disorder if diagnostic criteria are met. Coexisting mental and physical disorders are listed, but without the use of terms such as *related to* or *due to,* which were used in DSM-IV. Such terms imply a causal relationship, which often cannot be established. By avoiding etiological assumptions, the classification system reminds clinicians that insomnia disorder usually requires independent clinical attention in addition to management of coexisting mental and physical disorders. The changes also recognize the bidirectional and interactive effects between sleep disorders and coexisting medical and mental disorders.

The clinician confronted with complaints of sleep disturbance must define the nature of the complaint, whether primarily insomnia, excessive daytime sleepiness, dis-

---

TABLE 1.　　**DSM-5 sleep-wake disorders**

Insomnia disorder

Hypersomnolence disorder

Narcolepsy

Breathing-related sleep disorders

　Obstructive sleep apnea hypopnea

　Central sleep apnea

　Sleep-related hypoventilation

Circadian rhythm sleep-wake disorders

　Delayed sleep phase type

　Advanced sleep phase type

　Irregular sleep-wake type

　Non-24-hour sleep-wake type

　Shift work type

Parasomnias

　Non–rapid eye movement sleep arousal disorders

　　Sleepwalking type

　　Sleep terror type

　Nightmare disorder

　Rapid eye movement sleep behavior disorder

　Restless legs syndrome

Substance/medication-induced sleep disorder

Other specified insomnia disorder

Unspecified insomnia disorder

Other specified hypersomnolence disorder

Unspecified hypersomnolence disorder

Other specified sleep-wake disorder

Unspecified sleep-wake disorder

---

turbed mentation or behavior during sleep, or difficulties in the circadian placement of sleep. The first step in diagnosis should be to consider the individual's general medical condition, to determine whether the complaint represents a sleep disorder attributable to another medical condition. Furthermore, if the individual is taking a medication or using a substance, the clinician will need to consider the possibility of a substance/medication-induced sleep disorder.

If the main complaint is persistent insomnia and/or difficulty initiating or maintaining sleep, a diagnosis of insomnia disorder may be appropriate. If the primary complaint is excessive sleepiness, the clinician should consider the differential diagnosis of a hypersomnolence disorder, narcolepsy, or one of the breathing-related sleep disorders. If the individual frequently travels or is involved in shift work, or has a problem of sleep timing, a circadian rhythm sleep-wake disorder should be considered. If the individual's symptoms consist of predominantly behavioral or mental events during sleep (e.g., abrupt awakening, frightening dreams, or walking about while sleeping), the clinician should consider a diagnosis of an NREM sleep arousal disorder.

Insomnia Disorder

Insomnia, which is Latin for "no sleep," involves the predominant complaint of an inability to fall asleep or remain asleep. The word is also used to describe the condition of waking up not feeling restored or refreshed. Insomnia is the most common sleep complaint in the general population. It can be either acute (i.e., lasting one to several nights) or chronic (i.e., persisting for 1 month or longer). According to the National Center on Sleep Disorders Research at the National Institutes of Health, about 30%–40% of adults say they have symptoms of insomnia within a given year, and about 10%–15% of adults report chronic insomnia (National Institutes of Health 2005). Among individuals reporting chronic insomnia, most have chronic or intermittent symptoms, meaning that they experience difficulty sleeping for a few nights, followed by a few nights of adequate sleep before the problem returns.

Among those who report insomnia, sleep maintenance insomnia is the most frequent problem, followed by difficulty falling asleep and then early morning awakening. Complaints of poor sleep or insomnia increase with age, paralleling age-related changes in sleep-stage physiology. Young people with insomnia more frequently report difficulty falling asleep, whereas older individuals report middle and terminal insomnia. Furthermore, women of all ages report more sleep problems than men. Despite the large number of people with insomnia complaints, relatively few seek medical attention.

Insomnia can be a disorder in its own right or a symptom of another condition. Stress and worry are frequently blamed for insomnia. Insomnia can also occur with jet lag, shift work, and other major schedule changes. Research has consistently found a robust association between insomnia and psychiatric disorders—particularly depression and anxiety—across the life cycle. Persistent sleep disturbance was identified in the Epidemiologic Catchment Area study as a highly significant risk factor for the *subsequent* development of major depressive disorder (Ford and Kamerow 1989). Hence, early intervention to treat sleep disturbance might protect against depression.

Many changes have been made in the criteria for DSM-5 sleep-wake disorders. Three DSM-IV disorders—primary insomnia, insomnia related to another mental disorder, and sleep disorder due to a general medical condition, insomnia type—have been merged into the single DSM-5 diagnostic entity of insomnia disorder. The change moves away from the need to make causal attributions between co-occurring disorders, and acknowledges the interactive effects between sleep disorders and co-occurring medical or psychiatric conditions. Data show that in the majority of insomnia cases, the individual presents with another psychiatric or medical disorder, as opposed to the insomnia being a disorder on its own (i.e., primary insomnia in DSM-IV). Furthermore, the diagnostic reliability of insomnia, particularly primary insomnia, was relatively poor. Distinguishing between primary insomnia and insomnia due to a mental disorder or a medical condition was often difficult (or impossible), and the construct of secondary insomnia often led to undertreatment. In eliminating the distinction between primary and secondary insomnia, DSM-5 emphasizes that sleep disorders warrant independent clinical attention.

Diagnostic Criteria for Insomnia Disorder   **307.42** (F51.01)

A. A predominant complaint of dissatisfaction with sleep quantity or quality, associated with one (or more) of the following symptoms:
   1. Difficulty initiating sleep. (In children, this may manifest as difficulty initiating sleep without caregiver intervention.)
   2. Difficulty maintaining sleep, characterized by frequent awakenings or problems returning to sleep after awakenings. (In children, this may manifest as difficulty returning to sleep without caregiver intervention.)
   3. Early-morning awakening with inability to return to sleep.
B. The sleep disturbance causes clinically significant distress or impairment in social, occupational, educational, academic, behavioral, or other important areas of functioning.
C. The sleep difficulty occurs at least 3 nights per week.
D. The sleep difficulty is present for at least 3 months.
E. The sleep difficulty occurs despite adequate opportunity for sleep.
F. The insomnia is not better explained by and does not occur exclusively during the course of another sleep-wake disorder (e.g., narcolepsy, a breathing-related sleep disorder, a circadian rhythm sleep-wake disorder, a parasomnia).
G. The insomnia is not attributable to the physiological effects of a substance (e.g., a drug of abuse, a medication).
H. Coexisting mental disorders and medical conditions do not adequately explain the predominant complaint of insomnia.

Specify if:
   With non–sleep disorder mental comorbidity, including substance use disorders
   With other medical comorbidity
   With other sleep disorder

   Coding note: The code 780.52 (G47.00) applies to all three specifiers. Code also the relevant associated mental disorder, medical condition, or other sleep disorder immediately after the code for insomnia disorder in order to indicate the association.

Specify if:
   Episodic: Symptoms last at least 1 month but less than 3 months.
   Persistent: Symptoms last 3 months or longer.
   Recurrent: Two (or more) episodes within the space of 1 year.

Note: Acute and short-term insomnia (i.e., symptoms lasting less than 3 months but otherwise meeting all criteria with regard to frequency, intensity, distress, and/or impairment) should be coded as an other specified insomnia disorder.

Criterion A

DSM-5 has integrated the construct of sleep dissatisfaction into the definition of insomnia. Evidence suggests that the presence of sleep dissatisfaction in addition to insomnia symptoms increases considerably the proportion of individuals with daytime impairments relative to those with insomnia symptoms alone. Hence, adding sleep dissatisfaction to the definition of insomnia is likely to improve diagnostic specificity. This change could also improve detection of clinically significant insomnia among subgroups of individuals (e.g., older adults) who typically report little impairment or distress associated with insomnia symptoms but who are otherwise dissatisfied with their sleep. Criterion A requires dissatisfaction with quantity or quality regarding initiating sleep, maintaining sleep, or early morning awakenings. In addition, the criterion specifically highlights how these requirements may differ in children—that children may manifest difficulties initiating or maintaining sleep without caregiver intervention.

Criterion B

This criterion lists specific examples of the distress or impairments in daytime functioning resulting from insomnia. Many individuals with persistent insomnia (e.g., older adults) tend to minimize or underestimate the impact of insomnia on their daytime functioning, partly due to the lack of clear indicators of such impairments. This is likely to lead to underdiagnosis and absence of treatment. The addition of specific examples of impairments may enhance assessment and boost recognition of the impact of insomnia on daytime functioning.

Criteria C and D

Criterion C requires that the sleep disturbance be present for at least 3 nights each week (an addition in DSM-5). The minimum frequency criterion of 3 nights per week will differentiate individuals with occasional (subthreshold) insomnia from those with more clinically meaningful insomnia. Sensitivity and specificity indices are maximized (i.e., correct identification of true insomnia cases and correct exclusion of false positives), with a frequency of occurrence of insomnia falling between 3 and 4 nights per week. Also, this frequency criterion is consistent with that used in ICD-10 and with current research practices in the field. Evidence suggests that the frequency of occurrence of insomnia symptoms is an important determinant of morbidity and impairment.

The minimum duration of 3 months (Criterion D) reflects a change from the previous requirement of 1 month, which was a very short period to define insomnia as a chronic condition. By comparison, few psychiatric or medical conditions are considered chronic before they exceed 6- or 12-month durations. Insomnia lasting only 1 month might be better conceptualized as an *episode* rather than a disorder. Morbidity may also increase with insomnia persisting longer than 3 months.

Criterion E

This criterion requires that the sleep disturbance occur despite adequate opportunity for sleep. This criterion was added to help distinguish clinical insomnia from volitional sleep deprivation.

Criteria F, G, and H

These criteria are for ruling out other mental disorders and medical conditions. They indicate that the insomnia is not better explained by another sleep disorder, such as narcolepsy (or does not occur exclusively during the course of another sleep disorder); is not due to the effects of a substance (e.g., caffeine); and is not better explained by a coexisting medical condition or mental disorder.

Specifiers

Co-occurring mental health, substance use, and sleep disorders can be specified. In addition, there are three specifiers for the course of insomnia disorder: *episodic* (symptoms last at least 1 month but less than 3 months), *persistent* (symptoms last 3 months or longer), and *recurrent* (two or more episodes occur within the space of 1 year). Persistent insomnia is also associated with long-term consequences, including increased risks of major depressive disorder, hypertension, and myocardial infarction; increased absenteeism and reduced productivity at work; reduced quality of life; and increased economic burden.

Hypersomnolence Disorder

Excessive sleepiness poses a great challenge to the nearly one-third of adult Americans who report this problem (Ohayon et al. 2012). Although most healthy people require approximately 7 hours of sleep during the main sleep episode to feel refreshed and alert, many individuals curtail their sleep to meet social, vocational, or other demands. This exacts a high price, and many of these people struggle with excessive daytime sleepiness when they should be fully awake.

Excessive sleepiness can be associated with many sleep disorders, such as obstructive sleep apnea hypopnea, circadian rhythm sleep-wake disorders, and restless legs syndrome. It can also be induced by insomnia disorder, insufficient sleep, or poor sleep hygiene. When excessive sleepiness is associated with other symptoms, it qualifies for the diagnosis hypersomnolence disorder.

Dement et al. (1966) proposed that individuals with excessive daytime sleepiness, but without cataplexy, sleep paralysis, or sleep-onset REM periods, not be considered as having narcolepsy. Roth et al. (1972) later described a type of hypersomnia with sleep drunkenness that consists of difficulty coming to complete wakefulness, confusion, disorientation, poor motor coordination, and slowness, accompanied by deep and prolonged sleep. Abrupt sleep attacks seen in classic narcolepsy are not present in hypersomnolence disorder.

DSM-5 hypersomnolence disorder should be distinguished from excessive sleepiness related to insufficient sleep and from fatigue (tiredness not necessarily relieved by increased sleep and unrelated to sleep quantity or quality). Excessive sleepiness and fatigue are difficult to differentiate from hypersomnolence disorder and may overlap considerably. Individuals with this disorder have no difficulty falling asleep and have a sleep efficiency generally higher than 90%. They may experience confusional arousal upon awakening in the morning but also upon awakening from a daytime nap. During that period, the person appears awake but his or her behavior may be very inappropriate, with memory deficits, disorientation in time and space, and slow mentation and speech. The reduced vigilance and impaired cognitive response return to normal within 30–60 minutes (and sometimes longer). For some individuals with hypersomnolence disorder, the duration of the major sleep episode (nocturnal sleep for most individuals) is 9 hours or more. However, approximately 80% of individuals with a hypersomnolence disorder report their sleep as being nonrestorative, and just as many have difficulties awakening in the morning. Individuals with a hypersomnolence disorder may have daytime naps nearly every day regardless of the nocturnal sleep duration.

Several changes have been made from DSM-IV. DSM-5 has replaced the term *hypersomnia* with *hypersomnolence*. The disorder is characterized by a complaint of excessive sleepiness, which can be expressed in two main categories of symptoms: 1) excessive quantity of sleep, referring to extended nocturnal sleep or involuntary daytime sleep, and 2) deteriorated quality of wakefulness, referring to sleep propensity during wakefulness as shown by difficulty awakening or inability to remain awake when required. With DSM-IV, in many cases, severe excessive sleepiness symptoms remained undiagnosed because the excessive sleepiness was related to the quality of wakefulness, not the *quantity* of sleep. The term *hypersomnia* describes an excessive amount of sleep, whereas *hypersomnolence* refers to the main symptom of excessive sleepiness. Research shows that many individuals have excessive sleepiness that is not explained by another sleep disorder, but with normal amounts of sleep.

Epidemiological and clinical data indicate that individuals with hypersomnolence disorder often present with other psychiatric or medical conditions. DSM-5 has replaced three disorders—primary hypersomnia, hypersomnia related to another mental disorder, and sleep disorder due to a general medical condition, hypersomnia type—with a single diagnostic entity with specification of clinically comorbid conditions. The change in the terminology removes the need to make causal attributions between coexisting disorders and acknowledges the interactive effects of sleep disorders and coexisting medical and/or psychiatric disorders.

Diagnostic Criteria for Hypersomnolence Disorder   **307.44** (F51.11)

A. Self-reported excessive sleepiness (hypersomnolence) despite a main sleep period lasting at least 7 hours, with at least one of the following symptoms:
  1. Recurrent periods of sleep or lapses into sleep within the same day.
  2. A prolonged main sleep episode of more than 9 hours per day that is nonrestorative (i.e., unrefreshing).
  3. Difficulty being fully awake after abrupt awakening.
B. The hypersomnolence occurs at least three times per week, for at least 3 months.
C. The hypersomnolence is accompanied by significant distress or impairment in cognitive, social, occupational, or other important areas of functioning.
D. The hypersomnolence is not better explained by and does not occur exclusively during the course of another sleep disorder (e.g., narcolepsy, breathing-related sleep disorder, circadian rhythm sleep-wake disorder, or a parasomnia).

E. The hypersomnolence is not attributable to the physiological effects of a substance (e.g., a drug of abuse, a medication).

F. Coexisting mental and medical disorders do not adequately explain the predominant complaint of hypersomnolence.

Specify if:

With mental disorder, including substance use disorders

With medical condition

With another sleep disorder

Coding note: The code 780.54 (G47.10) applies to all three specifiers. Code also the relevant associated mental disorder, medical condition, or other sleep disorder immediately after the code for hypersomnolence disorder in order to indicate the association.

Specify if:

Acute: Duration of less than 1 month.

Subacute: Duration of 1–3 months.

Persistent: Duration of more than 3 months.

Specify current severity:

Specify severity based on degree of difficulty maintaining daytime alertness as manifested by the occurrence of multiple attacks of irresistible sleepiness within any given day occurring, for example, while sedentary, driving, visiting with friends, or working.

Mild: Difficulty maintaining daytime alertness 1–2 days/week.

Moderate: Difficulty maintaining daytime alertness 3–4 days/week.

Severe: Difficulty maintaining daytime alertness 5–7 days/week.

Criterion A

The clinical description of excessive sleepiness symptoms in DSM-IV was vague (i.e., complaint of excessive sleepiness "as evidenced by either prolonged sleep episodes or daytime sleep episodes that occur almost daily"). In many cases, severe excessive sleepiness symptoms remained undiagnosed because the excessive sleepiness was related to the *quality* of wakefulness, not the *quantity* of sleep. Additionally, in DSM-IV, no cut point was given to delineate what constituted a prolonged sleep episode. The threshold of 9 hours as indicative of a prolonged main sleep episode will help identify individuals with excessive amount of sleep. The choice of 9 hours was based on clinical evidence that individuals with hypersomnolence disorder (with or without long sleep time) sleep on average 8–8.5 hours on weekdays, and it represents the upper fifth percentile of the normal sleep distribution in the general population.

The DSM-IV symptom "daytime sleep episodes" has been refined: "Recurrent periods of sleep or lapses into sleep within the same day." This change allows for the inclusion of individuals who have a main sleep period of normal duration, defined as at least 7 hours of sleep, and have recurrent sleepiness episodes within the same day (at least two episodes). The duration of 7 hours was adopted because it is the average sleep duration of healthy adults, and it should reduce the possibility of including individuals whose excessive sleepiness might be due to insufficient sleep.

DSM-5 has added "difficulty being fully awake after abrupt awakening" as a core feature of excessive sleepiness. Difficulty in awakening from sleep is present in the majority of individuals (up to 78%) with hypersomnolence characterized by a long sleep time. Sleep inertia (sleep drunkenness) has been reported in 21%–72% of individuals with a hypersomnolence disorder. The addition of this symptom will increase precision in the identification of hypersomnolent individuals.

Criterion B

DSM-5 has added a minimum frequency criterion (i.e., three times per week) with excessive sleepiness. The frequency criterion (at least three times per week) was selected based on population data indicating that it was the best cutoff for sleepiness in terms of identifying individuals reporting impairment or distress associated with excessive sleepiness. The DSM-5 criterion replaces the "almost daily" requirement in DSM-IV and will help distinguish individuals with occasional sleepiness from those with more severe symptoms of excessive sleepiness.

DSM-5 also requires that the excessive sleepiness last at least 3 months. DSM-IV required a duration of 1 month, but that was perceived as too short a period to define excessive sleepiness as a chronic condition. Given that hypersomnolence disorder is generally a chronic condition, typically beginning in early adulthood, a time frame that reflects longer-term chronicity was chosen.

Criterion C

Irritability and cognitive dysfunction are frequent concerns of hypersomnolent individuals. Other symptoms may include anxiety, decreased energy, restlessness, slow speech, loss of appetite, and memory difficulties. Some individuals lose the ability to function in family, social, occupational, or other settings. Motor vehicle accidents are among the most serious of consequences stemming from excessive sleepiness. The National Sleep Foundation's (2005) Sleep in America poll indicated that 60% of behind-the-wheel adults have driven a motor vehicle while drowsy, and 13% have actually fallen asleep while driving at least once per month.

Criteria D, E, and F

Individuals with breathing-related sleep disorders may have patterns of excessive sleepiness, and circadian rhythm sleep-wake disorders are also often characterized by daytime sleepiness. Complaints of daytime sleepiness may occur with medical conditions (e.g., a major neurocognitive disorder), medications (e.g., antipsychotics), or mental disorders (e.g., during a major depressive episode or the depressed phase of bipolar disorder). A diagnosis of hypersomnolence disorder can be made in the presence of another current or past mental disorder as long as the other disorder does not completely explain the hypersomnolence.

Specifiers

The clinician may specify the presence of comorbid conditions: another mental disorder, including substance use disorders; another medical condition; and another sleep disorder. In each case, the specifier helps clarify the individual's condition.

In addition to the specifiers regarding co-occurring conditions, there are three specifiers available to describe course: *acute* (duration of less than 1 month), *subacute* (duration of 1–3 months), and *persistent* (duration of more than 3 months). Severity specifiers, based on difficulty maintaining daytime alertness, are included as well.

Narcolepsy

Narcolepsy is a disorder that leads to instability in the sleep-wake cycle. It causes excessive daytime sleepiness and leads to sudden onsets of REM sleep. Narcolepsy can put severe limitations on individuals' lives because of their inability to stay awake for long periods of time and because of the risk that accompanies sudden bouts of sleeping. It is a chronic condition that is treatable but not curable. Symptoms usually begin either between ages 15 and 25 years or between ages 30 and 35 years, but they can begin at any age. They include episodes of extreme drowsiness every 3–4 hours, dreamlike hallucinations, sleep paralysis, cataplexy (i.e., loss of all muscle tone in the body), and "sleep attacks" (i.e., short attacks triggered by varying conditions such as eating large meals, moments of high stress or tension, or being awake for more than 4 hours). Cataplexy can cause a person's head to drop or knees to buckle, or might cause the person to collapse in his or her seat or onto the floor, potentially leading to dangerous consequences.

The term *narcolepsy* was first used in 1880 by the French neurologist Gélineau, who used the term to describe a syndrome of recurrent, irresistible daytime sleep episodes, sometimes accompanied by sudden falls (Morin and Edinger 2009). The disorder was first included in DSM-IV and continues to be recognized in DSM-5. In the ICSD-2, both narcolepsy with catalepsy and narcolepsy without catalepsy are recognized as distinctive subtypes.

Evidence shows that narcolepsy is associated with a lowered amount of a protein called *hypocretin* in the brain. In the 1990s, hypocretin-2 gene deletions were found to be the disease mechanism in canine narcolepsy. In human studies, low levels of hypocretin-1 are found in the cerebrospinal fluid of narcolepsy patients, and losses of over 80% of hypocretin (orexin)–producing neurons in the dorsolateral hypothalamus have been reported in autopsy studies. One explanation might be that hypocretin-producing cells are destroyed by an autoimmune process.

Diagnostic Criteria for Narcolepsy

A. Recurrent periods of an irrepressible need to sleep, lapsing into sleep, or napping occurring within the same day. These must have been occurring at least three times per week over the past 3 months.

B. The presence of at least one of the following:

1. Episodes of cataplexy, defined as either (a) or (b), occurring at least a few times per month:

    a. In individuals with long-standing disease, brief (seconds to minutes) episodes of sudden bilateral loss of muscle tone with maintained consciousness that are precipitated by laughter or joking.

    b. In children or in individuals within 6 months of onset, spontaneous grimaces or jaw-opening episodes with tongue thrusting or a global hypotonia, without any obvious emotional triggers.

2. Hypocretin deficiency, as measured using cerebrospinal fluid (CSF) hypocretin-1 immunoreactivity values (less than or equal to one-third of values obtained in healthy subjects tested using the same assay, or less than or equal to 110 pg/mL). Low CSF levels of hypocretin-1 must not be observed in the context of acute brain injury, inflammation, or infection.

3. Nocturnal sleep polysomnography showing rapid eye movement (REM) sleep latency less than or equal to 15 minutes, or a multiple sleep latency test showing a mean sleep latency less than or equal to 8 minutes and two or more sleep-onset REM periods.

Specify whether:

347.00 (G47.419) Narcolepsy without cataplexy but with hypocretin deficiency: Criterion B requirements of low CSF hypocretin-1 levels and positive polysomnography/multiple sleep latency test are met, but no cataplexy is present (Criterion B1 not met).

347.01 (G47.411) Narcolepsy with cataplexy but without hypocretin deficiency: In this rare subtype (less than 5% of narcolepsy cases), Criterion B requirements of cataplexy and positive polysomnography/multiple sleep latency test are met, but CSF hypocretin-1 levels are normal (Criterion B2 not met).

347.00 (G47.419) Autosomal dominant cerebellar ataxia, deafness, and narcolepsy: This subtype is caused by exon 21 DNA (cytosine-5)-methyltransferase-1 mutations and is characterized by late-onset (age 30–40 years) narcolepsy (with low or intermediate CSF hypocretin-1 levels), deafness, cerebellar ataxia, and eventually dementia.

347.00 (G47.419) Autosomal dominant narcolepsy, obesity, and type 2 diabetes: Narcolepsy, obesity, and type 2 diabetes and low CSF hypocretin-1 levels have been described in rare cases and are associated with a mutation in the myelin oligodendrocyte glycoprotein gene.

347.10 (G47.429) Narcolepsy secondary to another medical condition: This subtype is for narcolepsy that develops secondary to medical conditions that cause infectious (e.g., Whipple's disease, sarcoidosis), traumatic, or tumoral destruction of hypocretin neurons.

Coding note (for ICD-9-CM code 347.10 only): Code first the underlying medical condition (e.g., 040.2 Whipple's disease; 347.10 narcolepsy secondary to Whipple's disease).

Specify current severity:

Mild: Infrequent cataplexy (less than once per week), need for naps only once or twice per day, and less disturbed nocturnal sleep.

Moderate: Cataplexy once daily or every few days, disturbed nocturnal sleep, and need for multiple naps daily.

Severe: Drug-resistant cataplexy with multiple attacks daily, nearly constant sleepiness, and disturbed nocturnal sleep (i.e., movements, insomnia, and vivid dreaming).

Criterion A

The wording of Criterion A has been changed from "Irresistible attacks of refreshing sleep that occur daily over at least 3 months" to focus on recurrent periods of an irrepressible need to sleep, lapses into sleep, or naps, occurring at least three times per week over the previous 3 months (when the individual is untreated).

Criterion B

In DSM-IV, only one of two criteria had to be met. In this revision, at least one of three criteria has to be met. Narcolepsy was originally described with the presence of cataplexy. Cataplexy is usually triggered by strong emotions, but studies have shown the type of emotions is more important than the intensity. Interestingly, joking is the most specific trigger that distinguishes true cataplexy in individuals with narcolepsy from other experiences reported by individuals without narcolepsy. Laughter is also commonly involved, although it may be more culturally dependent because mirth is the true trigger. In addition, cataplexy is almost always brief, and fewer than 15% of patients report that their attacks last longer than 2 minutes. From 5% to 10% of persons report having one attack per year (or fewer), and less than 20% report having attacks at least monthly (Dauvilliers et al. 2007). For this reason, several attacks per month is considered a reasonable frequency. For young children, the disorder may have a rapid onset that can occur over a few weeks. In these cases, cataplexy manifests differently, by semiconstant, tic-like partial hypotonia of the jaw with tongue protrusion or even a generalized weakness without a clear trigger. These rare cases evolve into the more classic form (with usual trigger) within 6 months to 1 year.

The finding of low cerebrospinal fluid (CSF) hypocretin-1 levels in individuals with narcolepsy has been replicated by investigators around the world. The particular threshold of less than or equal to one-third of mean control values, or ≤110 pg/mL, has been established by quantitative ROC (receiver operating characteristic) curves comparing samples drawn from individuals with narcolepsy with samples from healthy controls, patients with other sleep disorders (including narcolepsy without cataplexy, hypersomnia, insomnia), and patients with various acute or chronic neurological conditions (Burgess and Scammell 2012). Additionally, normal subjects essentially never have low CSF hypocretin levels, but some patients with severe acute neurological disorders (e.g., acute meningitis, severe head trauma) can have decreased CSF hypocretin, a finding that is reversible when or if the condition improves. Narcolepsy with cataplexy is almost always caused by hypocretin deficiency. Almost all patients with cataplexy have low or undetectable levels of hypocretin-1 in the CSF. In contrast, only 5%–30% of cases without cataplexy have low CSF hypocretin-1 levels.

In the late 1950s, it was discovered that individuals with narcolepsy also have a short REM sleep latency, a finding that led to using the multiple sleep latency test (MSLT) as a diagnostic test for narcolepsy (nocturnal sleep polysomnography showing mean sleep latency ≤15 minutes or, more recently, MSLT showing mean sleep latency ≤8 minutes with ≥2 sleep-onset REM periods in 4–5 naps as a positive test). The MSLT for narcolepsy-cataplexy has shown about 95% sensitivity and specificity, both when cataplexy is used as a gold standard and when CSF hypocretin has been measured. Research shows that the observation of a short REM latency during a nocturnal sleep study is more specific (~99%) but less sensitive (~50%) than a positive MSLT result (Andlauer et al. 2013). Sleep test criteria consistent with narcolepsy can be either a sleep-onset REM period at night (i.e., REM sleep latency ≤15 minutes) or a positive MSLT finding.

Subtypes and Specifiers

The subtypes allow the clinician to be more specific about causation by pinpointing the relationship of narcolepsy to hypocretin deficiency, chromosome 21 mutations, type 2 diabetes mellitus, neurological disorders, or an infectious cause. Current severity (mild, moderate, severe) may also be specified.

Breathing-Related Sleep Disorders

Rather than having a single set of criteria for breathing-related sleep disorder, as provided in DSM-IV, DSM-5 provides specific diagnostic criteria for a spectrum of breathing-related sleep disorders: obstructive sleep apnea hypopnea, central sleep apnea, and sleep-related hypoventilation. Although these disorders may share common underlying physiological risk factors (respiratory control instability), physiological and anatomical studies indicate differences in the pathogenesis of these disorders, with central sleep apnea less dependent on structural airway abnormalities as compared with obstructive sleep apnea, which is more dependent on increased upper airway resistance, and sleep-related hypoventilation, which is often comorbid with other disorders that depress ventilation. DSM-5 provides an overview of these interrelated disorders and specific definitions for each of these entities.

Obstructive Sleep Apnea Hypopnea

Obstructive sleep apnea hypopnea is the most common category of breathing-related sleep disorders. It is a potentially serious disorder in which breathing repeatedly stops and starts during sleep. A pause in breathing (and therefore total absence of airflow) is called an *apnea* episode. A decrease in airflow during breathing is called a *hypopnea* episode. Almost everyone has brief apnea episodes during sleep. The person with obstructive sleep apnea hypopnea is rarely aware of having difficulty breathing, even upon awakening. When the muscles relax, a person's airway narrows or closes as he or she breathes in, and breathing may be inadequate for 10–20 seconds. This period of inadequate breathing may lower the level of oxygen in the blood. The brain senses this impaired breathing and briefly rouses the person from sleep.

The most noticeable sign of obstructive sleep apnea hypopnea is *snoring.* This is recognized as a problem by others witnessing the individual during sleep episodes or is suspected because of its effects on the body. Because the muscle tone of the body ordinarily relaxes during sleep, and the airway at the throat is composed of walls of soft tissue, which can collapse, it is not surprising that breathing can be obstructed during sleep. Although a very minor degree of obstructive sleep apnea hypopnea is considered to be within the bounds of normal sleep, and many individuals experience episodes of obstructive sleep apnea at some point in life, only a small percentage of people are afflicted with chronic, severe obstructive sleep apnea hypopnea.

Obstructive sleep apnea hypopnea most commonly affects middle-age and older adults and people who are overweight. Signs and symptoms of obstructive sleep apnea hypopnea include excessive daytime sleepiness (hypersomnia), loud snoring, observed episodes of breathing cessation during sleep, abrupt awakenings accompanied by shortness of breath, awakening with a dry mouth or sore throat, morning headache, difficulty staying asleep (insomnia), and difficult-to-control high blood pressure. The breathing disruptions impair the ability to reach the desired deep, restful phases of sleep, resulting in sleepiness during waking hours. Diagnosis is based on polysomnographic findings and on symptoms.

Diagnostic Criteria for Obstructive Sleep Apnea Hypopnea   **327.23** (G47.33)

A. Either (1) or (2):

1. Evidence by polysomnography of at least five obstructive apneas or hypopneas per hour of sleep and either of the following sleep symptoms:

   a. Nocturnal breathing disturbances: snoring, snorting/gasping, or breathing pauses during sleep.

   b. Daytime sleepiness, fatigue, or unrefreshing sleep despite sufficient opportunities to sleep that is not better explained by another mental disorder (including a sleep disorder) and is not attributable to another medical condition.

2. Evidence by polysomnography of 15 or more obstructive apneas and/or hypopneas per hour of sleep regardless of accompanying symptoms.

Specify current severity:
   Mild: Apnea hypopnea index is less than 15.
   Moderate: Apnea hypopnea index is 15–30.
   Severe: Apnea hypopnea index is greater than 30.

Criterion A

DSM-5 includes symptoms of nocturnal breathing disturbances in the diagnostic criteria for obstructive sleep apnea hypopnea. Nocturnal symptoms reflect the occurrence of breathing disorders during the sleep period. Objective measurements of snoring intensity correlate with apnea hypopnea index. Snoring and gasping contribute significantly to sleep apnea prediction and in some studies are the most significant symptoms associated with sleep apnea. DSM-5 also includes polysomnographic criteria in the diagnostic criteria. Symptom reports are not sufficiently sensitive or specific to diagnose breathing-related sleep disorders, although they can be used as screening tools.

Specifiers

The severity of obstructive sleep apnea hypopnea is delineated based on an apnea hypopnea index (i.e., the number of apneas plus hypopneas per hour of sleep, as determined by polysomnography or other overnight monitoring). The disorder is mild if the index is less than 15, moderate if the index is between 15 and 30, and severe if the index is greater than 30. Regardless of the apnea hypopnea index, the disorder is considered to be more severe when apneas and hypopneas are accompanied by significant oxygen hemoglobin desaturation or when sleep is severely fragmented as shown by an elevated arousal index (arousal index greater than 30) or reduced stages in deep sleep.

Central Sleep Apnea

Central sleep apnea is a disorder in which breathing repeatedly stops and starts during sleep. It occurs because the brain fails to send proper signals to the muscles that control breathing. In contrast, in obstructive sleep apnea hypopnea, a person cannot breathe normally because of upper airway obstruction. Central sleep apnea is less common, accounting for fewer than 5% of sleep apnea cases.

Common signs and symptoms of central sleep apnea include observed episodes of stopped breathing or abnormal breathing patterns during sleep, abrupt awakenings accompanied by shortness of breath, shortness of breath relieved by sitting up, difficulty staying asleep (insomnia), excessive daytime sleepiness (hypersomnia), difficulty concentrating, morning headaches, and snoring. Although snoring indicates some degree of increased obstruction of airflow, snoring may also be heard in the presence of central sleep apnea; however, snoring may not be as prominent with central sleep apnea as it is with obstructive sleep apnea hypopnea. Central sleep apnea is associated with several conditions, including heart failure and chronic opioid use.

In DSM-IV, central sleep apnea was included in the breathing-related sleep disorder diagnosis and did not have separate criteria. Specific diagnostic criteria for central sleep apnea have been developed for DSM-5.

Diagnostic Criteria for Central Sleep Apnea

A. Evidence by polysomnography of five or more central apneas per hour of sleep.

B. The disorder is not better explained by another current sleep disorder.

Specify whether:

327.21 (G47.31) Idiopathic central sleep apnea: Characterized by repeated episodes of apneas and hypopneas during sleep caused by variability in respiratory effort but without evidence of airway obstruction.

786.04 (R06.3) Cheyne-Stokes breathing: A pattern of periodic crescendo-decrescendo variation in tidal volume that results in central apneas and hypopneas at a frequency of at least five events per hour, accompanied by frequent arousal.

780.57 (G47.37) Central sleep apnea comorbid with opioid use: The pathogenesis of this subtype is attributed to the effects of opioids on the respiratory rhythm generators in the medulla as well as the differential effects on hypoxic versus hypercapnic respiratory drive.

Coding note (for 780.57 [G47.37] code only): When an opioid use disorder is present, first code the opioid use disorder: 305.50 (F11.10) mild opioid use disorder or 304.00 (F11.20) moderate or severe opioid use disorder; then code 780.57 (G47.37) central sleep apnea comorbid with opioid use. When an opioid use disorder is not present (e.g., after a one-time heavy use of the substance), code only 780.57 (G47.37) central sleep apnea comorbid with opioid use.

Note: See the section "Diagnostic Features" in DSM-5 text.

Specify current severity:

Severity of central sleep apnea is graded according to the frequency of the breathing disturbances as well as the extent of associated oxygen desaturation and sleep fragmentation that occur as a consequence of repetitive respiratory disturbances.

Criteria A and B

Apnea episodes require polysomnographic data indicating five or more central apneas per hour of sleep. Clinical symptoms are not sufficiently sensitive or specific to diagnose central sleep apnea, although they can be used as a screening tool. Other sleep disorders need to be ruled out as a cause of the disturbance.

Subtypes and Specifiers

Clinicians may indicate if 1) the disorder is idiopathic and unrelated to airway obstruction, 2) a Cheyne-Stokes breathing pattern is present (characterized by a pattern of periodic crescendo-decrescendo variation in tidal volume that results in central apneas and hypopneas occurring at a frequency of at least five events per hour that are accompanied by frequent arousals), or 3) the disorder appears to be comorbid with opioid use. Current severity may also be recorded.

Sleep-Related Hypoventilation

Sleep-related hypoventilation is the result of decreased respiration associated with elevated carbon dioxide levels during sleep. Sleep-related hypoventilation is characterized by frequent episodes of shallow breathing lasting longer than 10 seconds during sleep. It is frequently associated with lung disease or neuromuscular or chest wall disorders, or medication use.

DSM-5 provides specific diagnostic criteria for sleep-related hypoventilation rather than, as in DSM-IV, incorporating the condition within the single criteria set for breathing-related sleep disorder. Although breathing-related sleep disorders may share common underlying physiological risk factors (respiratory control instability), physiological and anatomical studies indicate differences in the pathogenesis of these disorders, with sleep-related hypoventilation often comorbid with other disorders that depress ventilation.

Diagnostic Criteria for Sleep-Related Hypoventilation

A. Polysomnograpy demonstrates episodes of decreased respiration associated with elevated CO_2 levels. (**Note:** In the absence of objective measurement of CO_2, persistent low levels of hemoglobin oxygen saturation unassociated with apneic/hypopneic events may indicate hypoventilation.)

B. The disturbance is not better explained by another current sleep disorder.

Specify whether:

327.24 (G47.34) Idiopathic hypoventilation: This subtype is not attributable to any readily identified condition.

327.25 (G47.35) Congenital central alveolar hypoventilation: This subtype is a rare congenital disorder in which the individual typically presents in the perinatal period with shallow breathing, or cyanosis and apnea during sleep.

327.26 (G47.36) Comorbid sleep-related hypoventilation: This subtype occurs as a consequence of a medical condition, such as a pulmonary disorder (e.g., interstitial lung disease, chronic obstructive pulmonary disease) or a neuromuscular or chest wall disorder (e.g., muscular dystrophies, postpolio syndrome, cervical spinal cord injury, kyphoscoliosis), or medications (e.g., benzodiazepines, opiates). It also occurs with obesity (obesity hypoventilation disorder), where it reflects a combination of increased work of breathing due to reduced chest wall compliance and ventilation-perfusion mismatch and variably reduced ventilatory drive. Such individuals usually are characterized by body mass index of greater than 30 and hypercapnia during wakefulness (with a pCO_2 of greater than 45), without other evidence of hypoventilation.

Specify current severity:

Severity is graded according to the degree of hypoxemia and hypercarbia present during sleep and evidence of end organ impairment due to these abnormalities (e.g., right-sided heart failure). The presence of blood gas abnormalities during wakefulness is an indicator of greater severity.

Criteria A and B

As is the case for the other sleep disorders, specific polysomnographic findings are required for the diagnosis. Other sleep disorders need to be ruled out before making this diagnosis.

Subtypes and Specifiers

The clinician can record whether the hypoventilation is idiopathic, attributable to the rare congenital central alveolar hypoventilation syndrome (which presents in the perinatal period with shallow breathing, or cyanosis and apnea during sleep), or attributable to a comorbid disorder such as a pulmonary disease. Current severity may be indicated as well.

Circadian Rhythm Sleep-Wake Disorders

Circadian Rhythm Sleep-Wake Disorders

Human beings have biological rhythms known as *circadian rhythms* that are controlled by a biological clock and that work on a daily time scale. The rhythms affect body temperature, alertness, appetite, and hormone secretion, as well as sleep timing. Because of a person's circadian clock, sleepiness does not continuously increase as time passes. A person's desire and ability to fall asleep are influenced both by the length of time since the person woke from an adequate sleep and by internal circadian rhythms. Thus, the body is ready for sleep and for wakefulness at different times of the day.

A circadian rhythm sleep-wake disorder is a persistent or recurring pattern of sleep disruption resulting either from an altered sleep-wake schedule or from an inequality between a person's natural sleep-wake cycle and the sleep-related demands placed on him or her. The term *circadian rhythm* refers to a person's internal sleep- and wake-related rhythms that occur throughout a 24-hour period. The sleep disruption leads to insomnia or excessive sleepiness during the day, resulting in impaired functioning. People with circadian rhythm sleep-wake disorders are unable to sleep and wake at the times required for normal work, school, and social needs; however, they are generally able to get enough sleep if allowed to sleep and wake at the times dictated by their body clocks. Unless they also have another sleep disorder, their sleep is of normal quality.

DSM-5 circadian rhythm sleep-wake disorder criteria differ from DSM-IV in two notable areas. First, the name has changed from "circadian rhythm sleep disorders." Although it is well appreciated that individuals with circadian rhythm sleep-wake disorders have difficulty initiating and/or maintaining sleep, they also prominently suffer from impairment of wakefulness and often seek treatment for excessive sleepiness. Thus, the term *sleep-wake* captures the daytime and nighttime impairments in function that are characteristic of circadian dysfunction. Second, specifiers have been revised, as described later in this section.

Diagnostic Criteria for Circadian Rhythm Sleep-Wake Disorders

A. A persistent or recurrent pattern of sleep disruption that is primarily due to an alteration of the circadian system or to a misalignment between the endogenous circadian rhythm and the sleep–wake schedule required by an individual's physical environment or social or professional schedule.
B. The sleep disruption leads to excessive sleepiness or insomnia, or both.
C. The sleep disturbance causes clinically significant distress or impairment in social, occupational, and other important areas of functioning.

Coding note: For ICD-9-CM, code **307.45** for all subtypes. For ICD-10-CM, code is based on subtype.

Specify whether:
    307.45 (G47.21) Delayed sleep phase type: A pattern of delayed sleep onset and awakening times, with an inability to fall asleep and awaken at a desired or conventionally acceptable earlier time.

        Specify if:
        Familial: A family history of delayed sleep phase is present.

        Specify if:
        Overlapping with non-24-hour sleep-wake type: Delayed sleep phase type may overlap with another circadian rhythm sleep-wake disorder, non-24-hour sleep-wake type.

    307.45 (G47.22) Advanced sleep phase type: A pattern of advanced sleep onset and awakening times, with an inability to remain awake or asleep until the desired or conventionally acceptable later sleep or wake times.

        Specify if:
        Familial: A family history of advanced sleep phase is present.

    307.45 (G47.23) Irregular sleep-wake type: A temporally disorganized sleep-wake pattern, such that the timing of sleep and wake periods is variable throughout the 24-hour period.

    307.45 (G47.24) Non-24-hour sleep-wake type: A pattern of sleep-wake cycles that is not synchronized to the 24-hour environment, with a consistent daily drift (usually to later and later times) of sleep onset and wake times.

    307.45 (G47.26) Shift work type: Insomnia during the major sleep period and/or excessive sleepiness (including inadvertent sleep) during the major awake period associated with a shift work schedule (i.e., requiring unconventional work hours).

    307.45 (G47.20) Unspecified type

Specify if:
    Episodic: Symptoms last at least 1 month but less than 3 months.
    Persistent: Symptoms last 3 months or longer.
    Recurrent: Two or more episodes occur within the space of 1 year.

Criteria A, B, and C

The sleep disruption is primarily due to a circadian system alteration or a mismatch between the demands of the person's environment or work/social schedule and the person's internal circadian sleep-wake cycle. This mismatch leads to sleep disturbances, which in turn result in excessive sleepiness or insomnia, or both, as well as distress or functional impairment.

Subtypes and Specifiers

Subtypes include delayed sleep phase type, advanced sleep phase type, irregular sleep-wake type, non-24-hour sleep-wake type, and shift work type, as well as an unspecified type. The delayed sleep phase type may be further specified as familial or overlapping with non-24-hour sleep-wake type.

Delayed sleep phase type is based on a delay in the timing of the major sleep period (usually more than 2 hours) in relation to the desired sleep and wake times, resulting in difficulties waking in the morning and excessive sleepiness at work and impaired sleep at home.

The diagnosis of advanced sleep phase type is based primarily on a history of an advance in the timing of the major sleep period (usually more than 2 hours) in relation to the desired sleep and wake times, which results in symptoms of early morning insomnia and excessive daytime sleepiness. The rationale for inclusion of advanced sleep phase type was based on strong empirical evidence of earlier timing of circadian biomarkers, including melatonin and core body temperature rhythms, occurring 2–4 hours earlier than normal.

The diagnosis of irregular sleep-wake type is based primarily on a history of symptoms of insomnia at night (during the usual sleep period) and excessive sleepiness (napping) during the day. This type is characterized by a lack of discernible sleep-wake circadian rhythm. The individual has no major sleep period, and sleep is fragmented into at least three periods during the 24-hour day. In otherwise healthy subjects, the condition may be a result of very poor sleep hygiene; however, the irregular sleep-wake type is commonly associated with neurological impairment, such as developmental disability in children and dementia in older adults.

The diagnosis of non-24-hour sleep-wake type is based primarily on a history of symptoms of insomnia and/or excessive sleepiness due to lack of a stable entrainment or synchronization between the timing of the endogenous circadian rhythm and the 24-hour light-dark cycle. Individuals will typically present with periods of insomnia, excessive sleepiness, or both, alternating with asymptomatic periods. Starting with the asymptomatic period when the individual's sleep phase is aligned to the external environment, sleep latency will gradually increase and the individual will complain of sleep-onset insomnia. As the sleep phase continues to drift so that clock-drive for sleep is now in the daytime, individuals will have trouble staying awake during the day and complain of sleepiness, with subsequent negative impact on affect, cognition, and function. Because the circadian period is not aligned to the external 24-hour environment, symptoms will depend on when an individual tries to sleep in relation to the circadian rhythm of sleep propensity. The diagnosis of shift work type is based on a history of regularly scheduled work outside the daytime window of 8:00 A.M. to 6:00 P.M. This results in excessive sleepiness at work and impaired sleep at home.

The DSM-IV jet lag subtype has been dropped. The jet lag subtype was removed because travel across time zones typically involves transient or short-term impairments, and the sleep-wake dysfunction may represent normal physiology rather than a pathological response.

Parasomnias

Parasomnias are disorders characterized by abnormal behavioral, experiential, or physiological events occurring in association with sleep, specific sleep stages, or sleep-wake transitions.

Non–Rapid Eye Movement Sleep Arousal Disorders

The conditions making up the NREM sleep arousal disorders—sleepwalking and sleep terrors—represent variations of the simultaneous admixture of elements of both wakefulness and NREM sleep, a combination that results in the appearance of complex motor behavior without conscious awareness (sometimes called "state dissociation"). The overlap of these conditions in people and in animals is well established. The fact that human sleep can be characterized by the simultaneous coexistence of wake-like and sleeplike electroencephalographic patterns in different cortical areas supports the state-dissociation concept of NREM sleep arousal disorders.

Diagnostic Criteria for Non–Rapid Eye Movement Sleep Arousal Disorders

A. Recurrent episodes of incomplete awakening from sleep, usually occurring during the first third of the major sleep episode, accompanied by either one of the following:

1. **Sleepwalking:** Repeated episodes of rising from bed during sleep and walking about. While sleepwalking, the individual has a blank, staring face; is relatively unresponsive to the efforts of others to communicate with him or her; and can be awakened only with great difficulty.

2. **Sleep terrors:** Recurrent episodes of abrupt terror arousals from sleep, usually beginning with a panicky scream. There is intense fear and signs of autonomic arousal, such as mydriasis, tachycardia, rapid breathing, and sweating, during each episode. There is relative unresponsiveness to efforts of others to comfort the individual during the episodes.

B. No or little (e.g., only a single visual scene) dream imagery is recalled.

C. Amnesia for the episodes is present.

D. The episodes cause clinically significant distress or impairment in social, occupational, or other important areas of functioning.

E. The disturbance is not attributable to the physiological effects of a substance (e.g., a drug of abuse, a medication).

F. Coexisting mental and medical disorders do not explain the episodes of sleepwalking or sleep terrors.

Coding note: For ICD-9-CM, code **307.46** for all subtypes. For ICD-10-CM, code is based on subtype.

Specify whether:

307.46 (F51.3) Sleepwalking type

Specify if:

With sleep-related eating

With sleep-related sexual behavior (sexsomnia)

307.46 (F51.4) Sleep terror type

Criteria A, B, and C

NREM sleep arousal disorders are characterized by repeated episodes of incomplete arousals from sleep, usually beginning during the first third of the major sleep episode. The individual may *sleepwalk* (defined as repeated episodes of complex motor behavior initiated during sleep, including rising from bed and walking about) or experience *sleep terrors* (repeated occurrence of precipitous awakenings from sleep in abrupt terror, usually beginning with a panicky scream). If the individual awakens after these arousals, little or none of the dream or only fragmentary, single images are recalled and the person has amnesia for the episode.

Criteria D, E, and F

Consistent with other DSM-5 disorders, NREM sleep arousal disorders must be associated with clinically significant distress or impairment. The physiological effects of a substance (e.g., a drug of abuse, a medication) must be ruled out as a cause, as must coexisting other mental disorders and medical conditions.

Nightmare Disorder

Nightmare disorder is characterized by recurrent dreams that feel threatening or frightening or cause dysphoria. The person becomes fully oriented when awakened and can usually remember the dream. Because nightmares are relatively common in the general population, nightmare disorder should be considered only in cases where the nightmares are recurrent and result in significant distress or impairment.

Diagnostic Criteria for Nightmare Disorder   **307.47** (F51.5)

A. Repeated occurrences of extended, extremely dysphoric, and well-remembered dreams that usually involve efforts to avoid threats to survival, security, or physical integrity and that generally occur during the second half of the major sleep episode.
B. On awakening from the dysphoric dreams, the individual rapidly becomes oriented and alert.
C. The sleep disturbance causes clinically significant distress or impairment in social, occupational, or other important areas of functioning.
D. The nightmare symptoms are not attributable to the physiological effects of a substance (e.g., a drug of abuse, a medication).
E. Coexisting mental and medical disorders do not adequately explain the predominant complaint of dysphoric dreams.

Specify if:
   During sleep onset

Specify if:
   With associated non–sleep disorder, including substance use disorders
   With associated other medical condition
   With associated other sleep disorder

   Coding note: The code 307.47 (F51.5) applies to all three specifiers. Code also the relevant associated mental disorder, medical condition, or other sleep disorder immediately after the code for nightmare disorder in order to indicate the association.

Specify if:
   Acute: Duration of period of nightmares is 1 month or less.
   Subacute: Duration of period of nightmares is greater than 1 month but less than 6 months.
   Persistent: Duration of period of nightmares is 6 months or greater.

Specify current severity:
   Severity can be rated by the frequency with which the nightmares occur:
   Mild: Less than one episode per week on average.
   Moderate: One or more episodes per week but less than nightly.
   Severe: Episodes nightly.

Criteria A and B

DSM-5 has replaced "repeated awakenings" with "repeated occurrences." The change removes the requirement that nightmares awaken the individual and thereby removes the distinction made by some between nightmares (which cause awakenings) and bad dreams (which do not). The distress due to nightmares extends beyond the disruptions of nocturnal sleep that awakenings produce. First, up to 36% of chronic and 56% of acute nightmare patients report not suffering from awakenings from sleep, whereas as few as 11% claim that their nightmares always awaken them. Second, 69% of patients with nightmare disorder report having had at least one (nonawakening) bad dream whose emotional intensity is of equal or greater magnitude than that reported for their nightmares. For 22% of individuals, mean intensity ratings for their bad dreams equal or exceed mean intensity ratings for their nightmares (Hasler and Germain 2009). Third, even the most unpleasant dreams do not necessarily awaken the sleeper; clinicians have described many individuals who dream of dying violently in their dreams without waking up. These findings together point to the existence of a substantial group of individuals who have extremely intense, disturbing dreams that do not awaken them. When nightmares terminate upon awakening, the person exhibits a rapid return to full alertness. Dysphoria may persist into wakefulness and contribute to difficulty returning to sleep and lasting daytime distress.

DSM-5 has also changed "extended and extremely frightening dreams, usually involving threats to survival, security, or self-esteem" to "extended, extremely dysphoric, and well-remembered dreams that usually involve efforts to avoid threats to survival, security, or physical integrity." Fear may be the most common emotion characterizing nightmares, but it is by no means the only one. Studies indicate that a variety of dysphoric emotions occur in nightmares, including anger, sadness, frustration, disgust, confusion, and guilt. In fact, 30% of nightmares and 51% of bad dreams contain primary emotions other than fear (Nielsen and Zadra 2010)

Criterion C

Nightmares cause more significant subjective distress than demonstrable social or occupational impairment. If nightmares result in frequent awakenings or sleep avoidance, however, individuals may experience excessive daytime sleepiness, poor concentration, depression, anxiety, or irritability. Some individuals with nightmare disorder minimize or underestimate the impact of nightmares on their functioning, partly due to the lack of clear indicators of such impairments. This could lead to underdiagnosis and undertreatment.

Criteria D and E

The nightmare symptoms are not attributable to the physiological effects of a substance. The term *attributable to* more accurately reflects the fact that the precise causality of the nightmares is not known. Other mental disorders (e.g., panic disorder) and medical conditions (e.g., nocturnal seizures) need to be ruled out as possible causes of the dysphoric dreams. Bereavement may also be a cause of the dreams.

Rapid Eye Movement Sleep Behavior Disorder

REM sleep behavior disorder in both human beings and animals is well established and has the potential to cause dramatic and potentially violent or injurious behavior arising from REM sleep. Seen in animal experiments in the 1960s, REM sleep behavior disorder was first described in humans in 1986. Since then, it has been identified as one of the major types of parasomnias, likely second only in prevalence to the NREM sleep arousal disorders. The clinical features, polysomnographic findings (present in nearly every case), and response to medication have been well characterized. REM sleep behavior disorder is one of the most important causes of sleep-related injurious or violent behavior.

The extraordinary relationship between REM sleep behavior disorder and neurodegenerative disorders (particularly Parkinson's disease, dementia with Lewy bodies, and multiple system atrophy) has been clearly established. At least 50% of individuals with REM sleep behavior disorder presenting in sleep clinics will eventually (often with a delay of over 10 years) develop one of these conditions. REM sleep behavior disorder may be more prevalent in psychiatric populations. In addition, iatrogenic REM sleep behavior disorder induced by medications commonly prescribed by psychiatrists, including tricyclic antidepressants, selective serotonin reuptake inhibitors, or serotonin-norepinephrine reuptake inhibitors, is becoming increasingly recognized.

Diagnostic Criteria for Rapid Eye Movement Sleep Behavior Disorder   327.42 (G47.52)

A. Repeated episodes of arousal during sleep associated with vocalization and/or complex motor behaviors.
B. These behaviors arise during rapid eye movement (REM) sleep and therefore usually occur more than 90 minutes after sleep onset, are more frequent during the later portions of the sleep period, and uncommonly occur during daytime naps.
C. Upon awakening from these episodes, the individual is completely awake, alert, and not confused or disoriented.
D. Either of the following:
   1. REM sleep without atonia on polysomnographic recording.
   2. A history suggestive of REM sleep behavior disorder and an established synucleinopathy diagnosis (e.g., Parkinson's disease, multiple system atrophy).
E. The behaviors cause clinically significant distress or impairment in social, occupational, or other important areas of functioning (which may include injury to self or the bed partner).
F. The disturbance is not attributable to the physiological effects of a substance (e.g., a drug of abuse, a medication) or another medical condition.
G. Coexisting mental and medical disorders do not explain the episodes.

Criteria A, B, C, and D

REM sleep behavior disorder is characterized by repeated episodes of arousal, often associated with vocalizations and/or complex motor behaviors, during REM sleep. These behaviors often reflect motor responses to the content of action-filled or violent dreams and have been referred to as "dream-enacting behaviors." These behaviors may be very bothersome to the individual and the bed partner and can result in significant injury (e.g., falling, jumping out of bed, punching, or kicking). These behaviors occur only during REM sleep. Upon awakening, the individual is immediately alert and oriented and can usually recall the dream content. Further, either 1) REM sleep without atonia on polysomnographic recording or 2) a history suggestive of REM sleep behavior disorder and an established synucleinopathy diagnosis (e.g., Parkinson's disease) is present.

Criteria E, F, and G

The diagnosis of REM sleep behavior disorder requires clinically significant distress or impairment. The physiological effects of a substance (e.g., a drug of abuse, a medication) or another medical condition must be ruled out as causing the disturbance, and coexisting mental or medical disorders must have also been ruled out as a cause.

Restless Legs Syndrome

Restless legs syndrome is a sensorimotor, neurological sleep disorder characterized by a desire to move the legs (or arms), usually associated with uncomfortable sensations typically described as creeping, crawling, tingling, burning, or itching. Symptoms are worse when the individual is at rest, and frequent movements of the legs occur in an effort to relieve the uncomfortable sensations. Symptoms are worse in the evening or night and in some individuals occur only in the evening or night. In DSM-5, restless legs syndrome has been elevated to disorder status. DSM-IV included a brief summary of restless legs syndrome within the broader category of dyssomnia not otherwise specified.

Restless legs syndrome is common, with prevalence rates from 2.7% to 7.2% (the lower rates reflecting the added requirement of at least moderate distress). Women are 1.5–2 times more likely than men to have restless legs syndrome (Allen et al. 2005).

Restless legs syndrome is associated with significant clinical and functional impairment. The disorder is well documented to be associated with reduced sleep time, sleep fragmentation, and reports of more sleep disturbance. Objective studies demonstrate significant, objective sleep abnormalities for individuals with restless legs syndrome, with increased latency to sleep and higher arousal index as the most consistent findings.

Diagnostic Criteria for Restless Legs Syndrome   **333.94** (G25.81)

A. An urge to move the legs, usually accompanied by or in response to uncomfortable and unpleasant sensations in the legs, characterized by all of the following:

1. The urge to move the legs begins or worsens during periods of rest or inactivity.
2. The urge to move the legs is partially or totally relieved by movement.
3. The urge to move the legs is worse in the evening or at night than during the day, or occurs only in the evening or at night.

B. The symptoms in Criterion A occur at least three times per week and have persisted for at least 3 months.

C. The symptoms in Criterion A are accompanied by significant distress or impairment in social, occupational, educational, academic, behavioral, or other important areas of functioning.

D. The symptoms in Criterion A are not attributable to another mental disorder or medical condition (e.g., arthritis, leg edema, peripheral ischemia, leg cramps) and are not better explained by a behavioral condition (e.g., positional discomfort, habitual foot tapping).

E. The symptoms are not attributable to the physiological effects of a drug of abuse or medication (e.g., akathisia).

Criteria A and B

Criteria A and B are in line with the essential diagnostic features as defined in DSM-IV and are compatible with descriptions in the literature. Urges to move the legs must occur at least three times per week over a 3-month period to qualify for the diagnosis. This helps ensure that the disorder is not simply a transient disturbance.

Criterion C

Restless legs syndrome must significantly affect functioning or cause distress. Although the impact of milder symptoms is not well characterized, people may complain of disruption in at least one activity of daily living, with half reporting a negative impact on mood and nearly half reporting lack of energy. The most common consequences of restless legs syndrome are sleep disturbances, including reduced sleep time and sleep fragmentation.

Criteria D and E

Symptoms of restless legs syndrome cannot be solely accounted for by another mental disorder or medical or behavioral condition or by medication effects. The differentiation of restless legs syndrome from other conditions is important because many people report some urge or need to move the legs while at rest and do not have the disorder. The most important mimics of restless legs syndrome are leg cramps, positional discomfort, arthralgias or arthritis, myalgias, positional ischemia (numbness), leg edema, peripheral neuropathy, radiculopathy, and habitual foot tapping. Muscle "knots" or cramps, relief with a single postural shift, limitation in joints, soreness on palpation, and other abnormalities on physical examination are not characteristic of the syndrome. Worsening at night and periodic limb movements are more common in restless legs syndrome than in medication-induced akathisia or peripheral neuropathy.

Substance/Medication-Induced Sleep Disorder

In DSM-5, substance- and medication-induced sleep disturbances are combined in a single category. The essential feature of substance/medication-induced sleep disorder is a prominent sleep disturbance judged to be primarily associated with the known effects of a substance of abuse or a medication. These disturbances are relatively common in clinical settings but are not always straightforward to diagnose, and they depend on several factors, including the type of substance (or medication), the individual's response to the agent, and the substance's pharmacology. For example, caffeine is one of the most common causes of disrupted sleep and needs to be ruled out as a cause in any investigation of insomnia. Depending on the substance, one of four subtypes of sleep disturbance may be reported: insomnia type, daytime sleepiness type, parasomnia type, and a mixed type for cases in which more than one type of sleep disturbance is present and none predominates.

DSM-5 has included tobacco-induced sleep disorder in the list of diagnoses. Empirical evidence indicates that nicotine may be a sleep-disturbing substance.

Diagnostic Criteria for Substance/Medication-Induced Sleep Disorder

A. A prominent and severe disturbance in sleep.

B. There is evidence from the history, physical examination, or laboratory findings of both (1) and (2):

1. The symptoms in Criterion A developed during or soon after substance intoxication or after withdrawal from or exposure to a medication.

2. The involved substance/medication is capable of producing the symptoms in Criterion A.

C. The disturbance is not better explained by a sleep disorder that is not substance/medication-induced. Such evidence of an independent sleep disorder could include the following:

The symptoms precede the onset of the substance/medication use; the symptoms persist for a substantial period of time (e.g., about 1 month) after the cessation of acute withdrawal or severe intoxication; or there is other evidence suggesting the existence of an independent non-substance/medication-induced sleep disorder (e.g., a history of recurrent non-substance/medication-related episodes).

D. The disturbance does not occur exclusively during the course of a delirium.

E. The disturbance causes clinically significant distress or impairment in social, occupational, or other important areas of functioning.

Note: This diagnosis should be made instead of a diagnosis of substance intoxication or substance withdrawal only when the symptoms in Criterion A predominate in the clinical picture and when they are sufficiently severe to warrant clinical attention.

Coding note: The ICD-9-CM and ICD-10-CM codes for the [specific substance/medication]-induced sleep disorders are indicated in the table below. Note that the ICD-10-CM code depends on whether or not there is a comorbid substance use disorder present for the same class of substance. If a mild substance use disorder is comorbid with the substance-induced sleep disorder, the 4th position character is "1," and the clinician should record "mild [substance] use disorder" before the substance-induced sleep disorder (e.g., "mild cocaine use disorder with cocaine-induced sleep disorder"). If a moderate or severe substance use disorder is comorbid with the substance-induced sleep disorder, the 4th position character is "2," and the clinician should record "moderate [substance] use disorder" or "severe [substance] use disorder," depending on the severity of the comorbid substance use disorder. If there is no comorbid substance use disorder (e.g., after a one-time heavy use of the substance), then the 4th position character is "9," and the clinician should record only the substance-induced sleep disorder. A moderate or severe tobacco use disorder is required in order to code a tobacco-induced sleep disorder; it is not permissible to code a comorbid mild tobacco use disorder or no tobacco use disorder with a tobacco-induced sleep disorder.

		ICD-10-CM		
	ICD-9-CM	With use disorder, mild	With use disorder, moderate or severe	Without use disorder
Alcohol	291.82	F10.182	F10.282	F10.982
Caffeine	292.85	F15.182	F15.282	F15.982
Cannabis	292.85	F12.188	F12.288	F12.988
Opioid	292.85	F11.182	F11.282	F11.982
Sedative, hypnotic, or anxiolytic	292.85	F13.182	F13.282	F13.982
Amphetamine (or other stimulant)	292.85	F15.182	F15.282	F15.982
Cocaine	292.85	F14.182	F14.282	F14.982
Tobacco	292.85	NA	F17.208	NA
Other (or unknown) substance	292.85	F19.182	F19.282	F19.982

Specify whether:

Insomnia type: Characterized by difficulty falling asleep or maintaining sleep, frequent nocturnal awakenings, or nonrestorative sleep.

Daytime sleepiness type: Characterized by predominant complaint of excessive sleepiness/fatigue during waking hours or, less commonly, a long sleep period.

Parasomnia type: Characterized by abnormal behavioral events during sleep.

Mixed type: Characterized by a substance/medication-induced sleep problem characterized by multiple types of sleep symptoms, but no symptom clearly predominates.

Specify if (see Table 1 in the chapter "Substance-Related and Addictive Disorders" [in DSM-5] for diagnoses associated with substance class):

With onset during intoxication: This specifier should be used if criteria are met for intoxication with the substance/medication and symptoms developed during the intoxication period.

With onset during discontinuation/withdrawal: This specifier should be used if criteria are met for discontinuation/withdrawal from the substance/medication and symptoms developed during, or shortly after, discontinuation of the substance/medication.

Criteria A and B

The criteria require that the sleep disturbance be severe. This limits the diagnosis to sleep problems that merit independent clinical attention. The criteria further require that one can attribute the sleep disturbance to the pharmacological effects of the substance.

Criterion C

Criterion C requires that the disturbance not be better accounted for by a sleep disorder that is not induced by a substance or medication. Evidence could include the following: 1) symptoms precede onset of the substance or medication use; 2) symptoms persist for a substantial period of time (e.g., about 1 month) after the cessation of acute withdrawal or severe intoxication; or 3) there is other evidence suggesting the existence of an independent non-substance/medication-induced sleep disorder (e.g., a history of recurrent non-substance/medication-related episodes).

Criterion D

If the sleep disturbance occurs only during the course of a delirium, it should not warrant a separate diagnosis.

Criterion E

The sleep disturbance from the substance needs to result in clinically significant distress or impairment. Increased risk for relapse is one unique functional consequence of this disorder.

Other Specified Insomnia Disorder and Unspecified Insomnia Disorder

These are residual categories to use for symptoms of an insomnia disorder that cause clinically significant distress or impairment but do not meet criteria for a more specific disorder in the class. The category other specified insomnia disorder is used when the clinician chooses to communicate the reason that the presentation does not meet full criteria. The clinician is encouraged to record the specific reason (e.g., brief insomnia disorder).

The category unspecified insomnia disorder is used when the clinician chooses *not* to specify the reason the criteria are not met, or there is insufficient information to make a more specific diagnosis.

Other Specified Insomnia Disorder   **780.52** (G47.09)

This category applies to presentations in which symptoms characteristic of insomnia disorder that cause clinically significant distress or impairment in social, occupational, or other important areas of functioning predominate but do not meet the full criteria for insomnia disorder or any of the disorders in the sleep-wake disorders diagnostic class. The other specified insomnia disorder category is used in situations in which the clinician chooses to communicate the specific reason that the presentation does not meet the criteria for insomnia disorder or any specific sleep-wake disorder. This is done by recording "other specified insomnia disorder" followed by the specific reason (e.g., "brief insomnia disorder").

Examples of presentations that can be specified using the "other specified" designation include the following:

1. **Brief insomnia disorder:** Duration is less than 3 months.
2. **Restricted to nonrestorative sleep:** Predominant complaint is nonrestorative sleep unaccompanied by other sleep symptoms such as difficulty falling asleep or remaining asleep.

Unspecified Insomnia Disorder   780.52 (G47.00)

This category applies to presentations in which symptoms characteristic of insomnia disorder that cause clinically significant distress or impairment in social, occupational, or other important areas of functioning predominate but do not meet the full criteria for insomnia disorder or any of the disorders in the sleep-wake disorders diagnostic class. The unspecified insomnia disorder category is used in situations in which the clinician chooses *not* to specify the reason that the criteria are not met for insomnia disorder or a specific sleep-wake disorder, and includes presentations in which there is insufficient information to make a more specific diagnosis.

Other Specified Hypersomnolence Disorder and Unspecified Hypersomnolence Disorder

These are residual categories to use for symptoms of a hypersomnolence disorder that cause clinically significant distress or impairment but do not meet criteria for a more specific disorder in the class. The category other specified hypersomnolence disorder is used when the clinician chooses to communicate the reason that the presentation does not meet full criteria. The clinician is encouraged to record the specific reason (e.g., brief-duration hypersomnolence).

The category unspecified hypersomnolence disorder is used when the clinician chooses *not* to specify the reason the criteria are not met, or there is insufficient information to make a more specific diagnosis.

Other Specified Hypersomnolence Disorder   780.54 (G47.19)

This category applies to presentations in which symptoms characteristic of hypersomnolence disorder that cause clinically significant distress or impairment in social, occupational, or other important areas of functioning predominate but do not meet the full criteria for hypersomnolence disorder or any of the disorders in the sleep-wake disorders diagnostic class. The other specified hypersomnolence disorder category is used in situations in which the clinician chooses to communicate the specific reason that the presentation does not meet the criteria for hypersomnolence disorder or any specific sleep-wake disorder. This is done by recording "other specified hypersomnolence disorder" followed by the specific reason (e.g., "brief-duration hypersomnolence," as in Kleine-Levin syndrome).

Unspecified Hypersomnolence Disorder   **780.54** (G47.10)

This category applies to presentations in which symptoms characteristic of hypersomnolence disorder that cause clinically significant distress or impairment in social, occupational, or other important areas of functioning predominate but do not meet the full criteria for hypersomnolence disorder or any of the disorders in the sleep-wake disorders diagnostic class. The unspecified hypersomnolence disorder category is used in situations in which the clinician chooses *not* to specify the reason that the criteria are not met for hypersomnolence disorder or a specific sleep-wake disorder, and includes presentations in which there is insufficient information to make a more specific diagnosis.

Other Specified Sleep-Wake Disorder and Unspecified Sleep-Wake Disorder

The other specified sleep-wake disorder category applies in situations in which symptoms characteristic of a sleep-wake disorder that cause clinically significant distress or functional impairment predominate but do not meet full criteria for any of the disorders in the sleep-wake disorders diagnostic class, and do not qualify for a diagnosis of other specified insomnia disorder or other specified hypersomnolence disorder.

The unspecified sleep-wake disorder category applies in situations in which the clinician chooses not to specify the reason that the criteria are not met for a specific sleep-wake disorder, or there is insufficient information to make a more specific diagnosis.

Other Specified Sleep-Wake Disorder   **780.59** (G47.8)

This category applies to presentations in which symptoms characteristic of a sleep-wake disorder that cause clinically significant distress or impairment in social, occupational, or other important areas of functioning predominate but do not meet the full criteria for any of the disorders in the sleep-wake disorders diagnostic class and do not qualify for a diagnosis of other specified insomnia disorder or other specified hypersomnolence disorder. The other specified sleep-wake disorder category is used in situations in which the clinician chooses to communicate the specific reason that the presentation does not meet the criteria for any specific sleep-wake disorder. This is done by recording "other specified sleep-wake disorder" followed by the specific reason (e.g., "repeated arousals during rapid eye movement sleep without polysomnography or history of Parkinson's disease or other synucleinopathy").

Unspecified Sleep-Wake Disorder   **780.59** (G47.9)

This category applies to presentations in which symptoms characteristic of a sleep-wake disorder that cause clinically significant distress or impairment in social, occupational, or other important areas of functioning predominate but do not meet the full criteria for any of the disorders in the sleep-wake disorders diagnostic class and do not qualify for a diagnosis of unspecified insomnia disorder or unspecified hypersomnolence disorder. The unspecified sleep-wake disorder category is used in situations in which the clinician chooses *not* to specify the reason that the criteria are not met for a specific sleep-wake disorder, and includes presentations in which there is insufficient information to make a more specific diagnosis.

Key Points

- The revision of the sleep disorders chapter for DSM-5 has been influenced by the second edition of the *International Classification of Sleep Disorders*, published by the American Academy of Sleep Medicine.

- The diagnosis primary insomnia has been renamed *insomnia disorder* to avoid the differentiation between primary and secondary insomnia. Narcolepsy—now known to be associated with hypocretin—is distinguished from other forms of hypersomnolence (hypersomnolence disorder).

- Breathing-related sleep disorders are divided into three distinct disorders: obstructive sleep apnea hypopnea, central sleep apnea, and sleep-related hypoventilation.

- The subtypes of circadian rhythm sleep disorders (now called *circadian rhythm sleep-wake disorders*) have been expanded to include advanced sleep phase type and irregular sleep-wake type, and the jet lag type has been omitted.

- Rapid eye movement sleep behavior disorder and restless legs syndrome have achieved independent disorder status. Both were included in DSM-IV as examples of a "not otherwise specified" diagnosis.

References

Allen RP, Walters AS, Montplaisir J, et al: Restless legs syndrome prevalence and impact: REST general population study. Arch Intern Med 165:1286–1292, 2005

Andlauer O, Moore H, Jouhier L, et al: Nocturnal rapid eye movement sleep latency for identifying patients with narcolepsy/hypocretin deficiency. JAMA Neurol 6:1–12, 2013

Burgess CR, Scammell TE: Narcolepsy: neural mechanisms of sleepiness and cataplexy. J Neurosci 32:12305–12311, 2012

Dauvilliers Y, Arnulf I, Mignot E: Narcolepsy with cataplexy. Lancet 369:499–511, 2007

Dement W, Rechtschaffen A, Gulevich G: The nature of the narcoleptic sleep attack. Neurology 16:18–33, 1966

Ford DE, Kamerow DB: Epidemiologic study of sleep disturbances and psychiatric disorders: an opportunity for prevention? JAMA 262:1479–1484, 1989

Hasler B, Germain A: Correlates and treatments of nightmares in adults. Sleep Med Clin 4:507–517, 2009

Morin CM, Edinger JD: Sleep/wake disorders, in Oxford Textbook of Psychopathology, 2nd Edition. Edited by Blaney PH, Millon T. New York, Oxford University Press, 2009, pp 506–526

National Institutes of Health: National Institutes of Health State of the Science Conference statement on Manifestations and Management of Chronic Insomnia in Adults, June 13–15, 2005. Sleep 28:1049–1057, 2005

National Sleep Foundation: 2005 adult sleep habits and styles (Sleep in America polls). Available at: http://www.sleepfoundation.org/article/sleep-america-polls/2005-adult-sleep-habits-and-styles. Accessed July 12, 2013.

Nielsen T, Zadra A: Idiopathic nightmares and dream disturbances associated with sleep-wake transitions, in Principles and Practice of Sleep Medicine, 5th Edition. Edited by Kryger MH, Roth T, Dement WC. New York, Elsevier, 2010, pp 1106–1115

Ohayon MM, Dauvilliers Y, Reynolds CF: Operational definitions and algorithms for excessive sleepiness in the general population: implications for DSM-5 nosology. Arch Gen Psychiatry 69:71–79, 2012

Roth B, Nevsimalova S, Rechtschaffen A: Hypersomnia with "sleep drunkenness." Arch Gen Psychiatry 26:456–462, 1972

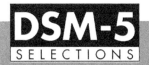

Sleep-Wake Disorders
DSM-5® Clinical Cases

Introduction

John W. Barnhill, M.D.

The pursuit of restful sleep is bedeviled by work and family pressures, long-distance travel, and the ubiquitous presence of stimulants (e.g., coffee) and electronics (e.g., e-mail). A good night's sleep can be a casualty of a host of psychiatric disorders, including anxiety, depression, and bipolar and psychotic disorders, as well as a variety of nonpsychiatric medical conditions. Sleep problems may not simply be epiphenomena but can precipitate, prolong, and intensify these other psychiatric and medical conditions. All too often, however, the DSM-5 sleep-wake disorders exist as silent and undiagnosed contributors to distress and dysfunction.

DSM-5 makes use of both a "lumping" and a "splitting" approach to the sleep disorders. Insomnia disorder can exist autonomously, but DSM-5 encourages consideration of comorbidity with both psychiatric and nonpsychiatric medical conditions. In so doing, DSM-5 moves away from making a causal attribution (e.g., depression inevitably causes insomnia) and instead acknowledges the bidirectional interactions between sleep and other disorders. Clarification of an independent sleep disorder is also a reminder to the clinician that the sleep problem may not resolve spontaneously but instead may warrant independent psychiatric attention.

In addition to a broad clinical approach, DSM-5 features sleep disorders that require very specific physiological findings. For example, a patient may present with restless sleep and daytime fatigue. If the patient's bed partner identifies unusually loud snoring, sleep apnea would likely be considered. A DSM-5 diagnosis of obstructive sleep apnea hypopnea requires not only clinical evidence but also a polysomnogram that reveals at least five obstructive apneas or hypopneas per hour of sleep (or, if there is no evidence of nocturnal breathing difficulties, 15 or more such apneic events per hour).

Other sleep disorders can be diagnosed through either clinical evidence or a combination of patient report, laboratory results, and sleep studies. For example, narcolepsy is defined by two required criteria. First, clinical report must indicate recurrent, persistent episodes marked by irrepressible sleep or an irrepressible need for sleep. The second criterion can be met in three ways: by recurrent episodes of cataplexy (defined clinically); hypocretin deficiency (defined via cerebrospinal fluid levels obtained through lumbar puncture); or specifically abnormal rapid eye movement

(REM) sleep latency as determined by nocturnal sleep polysomnography or a multiple sleep latency test.

REM sleep behavior disorder and restless legs syndrome are new disorders within the main text of DSM-5. For each, substantial evidence has clarified the physiological basis, prevalence, and clinical relevance. Both are often comorbid with other psychiatric and nonpsychiatric medical conditions (e.g., REM sleep behavior disorder comorbid with narcolepsy and neurodegenerative disorders such as Parkinson's disease; restless legs syndrome comorbid with depression and cardiovascular disease).

The initial sleep assessment generally involves a retrospective patient report. Clinicians are accustomed to working with subjective reports, but a sleep complaint that is impossible ("I haven't slept in weeks") can lead the clinician to think "insomnia" and move on with other aspects of the evaluation. Increasingly robust diagnostic criteria for the sleep-wake disorders are helpful for a variety of reasons, but they are especially helpful as a reminder to the general clinician to explore common complaints that are often underdiagnosed and that contribute to significant distress and dysfunction.

Suggested Readings

Edinger JD, Wyatt JK, Stepanski EJ, et al: Testing the reliability and validity of DSM-IV-TR and ICSD-2 insomnia diagnoses: results of a multitrait-multimethod analysis. Arch Gen Psychiatry 68(10):992–1002, 2011

Ohayon MM, Reynolds CF 3rd: Epidemiological and clinical relevance of insomnia diagnosis algorithms according to the DSM-IV and the International Classification of Sleep Disorders (ICSD). Sleep Med 10(9):952–960, 2009

Reite M, Weissberg M, Ruddy J: Clinical Manual for Evaluation and Treatment of Sleep Disorders. Washington, DC, American Psychiatric Publishing, 2009

Case 1: Difficulty Staying Asleep

Charles F. Reynolds III, M.D.

Aidan Jones, a 30-year-old graduate student in English, visited a psychiatrist to discuss his difficulty staying asleep. The trouble began 4 months earlier, when he started to wake up at 3:00 every morning, no matter when he went to bed, and then was unable to fall back to sleep. As a result, he felt "out of it" during the day. This led him to feel increasingly worried about how he was going to finish his doctoral dissertation when he was unable to concentrate owing to exhaustion. At first he did not recall waking up with anything in particular on his mind. As the trouble persisted, he found himself dreading the upcoming day and wondering how he would teach his classes or focus on his writing if he was getting only a few hours of sleep. Some mornings he lay awake in the dark next to his fiancée, who was sleeping soundly. On other mornings he would cut his losses, rise from bed, and go very early to his office on campus.

After a month of interrupted sleep, Mr. Jones visited a physician's assistant at the university's student health services, where he customarily got his medical care. (He suffered from asthma, for which he occasionally took inhaled β_2-adrenergic receptor agonists, and a year earlier he had had mononucleosis.) The physician's assistant prescribed a sedative-hypnotic, which did not help. "Falling asleep was never the problem," Mr. Jones explained. Meanwhile, he heeded some of the advice he read online. Although he felt reliant on coffee during the day, he never drank it after 2:00 P.M. An avid tennis player, he restricted his court time to the early morning. He did have a glass or two of wine every night at dinner with his fiancée, however. "By dinnertime I start to worry about whether I'll be able to sleep," he said, "and, to be honest, the wine helps."

The patient, a slender and fit-appearing young man looking very much the part of the young academic in a tweed jacket and tortoise-rimmed glasses, was pleasant and open in his storytelling. Mr. Jones did not appear tired but told the evaluating psychiatrist, "I made a point to see you in the morning, before I hit the wall." He did not look sad or on edge and was not sure if he had ever felt depressed. But he was certain of the nagging, low-level anxiety that was currently oppressing him. "This sleep problem has taken over," he explained. "I'm stressed about my work, and my fiancée and I have been arguing. But it's all because I'm so tired."

Although this was his first visit to a psychiatrist, Mr. Jones spoke of a fulfilling 3-year psychodynamic psychotherapy with a social worker while in college. "I was just looking to understand myself better," he explained, adding with a chuckle that as the son of a child psychiatrist, he was accustomed to people assuming he was "crazy." He recalled always being an "easy sleeper" prior to his recent difficulties; as a child he was the first to fall asleep at slumber parties, and as an adult he inspired the envy of his fiancée for the ease with which he could doze off on an airplane.

Diagnosis

• Insomnia disorder

Discussion

Mr. Jones reports 4 months of feeling dissatisfied with his sleep most nights, with difficulty maintaining sleep and early morning awakening. He describes daytime fatigue, difficulty concentrating, mild symptoms of anxiety, and interpersonal and vocational impairment. He does not appear to qualify for diagnoses of other medical, psychiatric, sleep, or substance use disorders. He meets the clinical criteria for DSM-5 insomnia disorder.

The case history suggests that the patient's sleep disturbance began during a period of heightened stress related to time pressures and that he has developed some behaviors that may worsen or perpetuate his sleep disturbance. He worries about not sleeping and creates a self-fulfilling prophecy. He may also be self-medicating with caffeine to maintain alertness during the day and with wine to dampen arousal during the evening.

Also noted is a medical history of asthma, for which Mr. Jones takes occasional β_2-adrenergic receptor agonists. Because these medications may be stimulating, it would be helpful to know when and how much of them he actually uses.

The patient reports a history of participating for 3 years in psychodynamic psychotherapy while in college. It would be helpful to know more about his mood and anxiety symptoms to determine whether his insomnia might be related to an earlier, and perhaps recurrent, mood or anxiety disorder. Conversely, insomnia itself increases the risk for either new-onset or recurrent episodes of mood, anxiety, or substance use disorders. It might also be helpful to explore Mr. Jones's family history of mood, anxiety, substance use, or sleep disorders.

A 2-week sleep-wake diary would be helpful in evaluating Mr. Jones's sleep issues, including the amount of time spent in bed, his lifestyle (timing of physical and mental activities that could increase arousal and interfere with sleep), the timing and use of substances that can act on the central nervous system, and other medical issues (e.g., asthma attacks). A history from Mr. Jones's fiancée could be informative with respect to his sleep-related pathologies, such as apnea, loud snoring, leg jerks, or partial arousals from sleep (non-REM or REM parasomnias).

In addition to having Mr. Jones keep a sleep-wake diary, it would be useful to have him document the severity of his current sleep complaint by use of a self-report inventory such as the Insomnia Severity Index (ISI) or the Pittsburgh Sleep Quality Index (PSQI). These instruments provide useful baselines or benchmarks against which to measure change over time. In addition, the use of brief self-report measures of affective state, such as the Patient Health Questionnaire 9-item depression scale (PHQ-9) or the Generalized Anxiety Disorder 7-item scale (GAD-7), would allow the clinician to further assess for coexisting or supervening mental disorders.

Formal sleep laboratory testing (polysomnography) does not appear to be indicated for Mr. Jones. However, if further information emerged from history or diary, it could be appropriate to obtain testing for a breathing-related sleep disorder or for periodic limb movement disorder. Another diagnostic possibility is a circadian rhythm sleep disorder, such as an advanced sleep phase syndrome (unlikely, however, given the relatively young age of the patient).

As illustrated by this case, DSM-5 has moved away from categorizing "primary" or "secondary" forms of insomnia disorder. Instead, DSM-5 mandates concurrent specification of coexisting conditions (medical, psychiatric, and other sleep disorders), for two reasons: 1) to underscore that the patient has a sleep disorder warranting independent clinical attention, in addition to the medical or psychiatric disorder also present, and 2) to acknowledge bidirectional and interactive effects between sleep disorders and coexisting medical and psychiatric disorders.

This reconceptualization reflects a paradigm shift in the field of sleep disorders medicine. The shift is away from making causal attributions between coexisting disorders ("a" is due to "b"), because there are often limited empirical data to support such attribution and because optimal treatment planning requires attention to both "a" and "b" (because the co-occurrence of each may make the other worse).

Thus, the differential diagnosis of sleep-wake complaints necessitates a multidimensional approach, with consideration of coexisting conditions. Such conditions are the rule, not the exception. Finally, the DSM-5 classification of insomnia disorder and other sleep-wake disorders includes dimensional as well as categorical assessment, for several reasons: 1) to capture severity, 2) to facilitate measurement-based clinical care, 3) to capture behaviors that may contribute to the pathogenesis and perpetuation of sleep-wake complaints, and 4) to allow correlation with and exploration of underlying neurobiological substrates.

Suggested Readings

Chapman DP, Presley-Cantrell LR, Liu Y, et al: Frequent insufficient sleep and anxiety and depressive disorders among U.S. community dwellers in 20 states, 2010. Psychiatr Serv 64(4):385–387, 2013

Reynolds CF 3rd: Troubled sleep, troubled minds, and DSM-5. Arch Gen Psychiatry 68(10):990–991, 2011

Reynolds CF 3rd, O'Hara R: DSM-5 sleep-wake disorders classification: overview for use in clinical practice. Am J Psychiatry 170(10):1099–1101, 2013

Case 2: Anxious and Sleepy

Maurice M. Ohayon, M.D., D.Sc., Ph.D.

Bernadette Kleber was a 34-year-old divorced, unemployed white mother of three school-age children. She was living with a new companion. Ms. Kleber presented to a psychiatrist for anxiety and sleepiness.

Ms. Kleber had experienced anxiety much of her life, but she had become much more worried and stressed since the birth of her first child 10 years before. She said she was "okay at home" but anxious in social situations. She avoided having to interact with new people, fearing that she would be embarrassed and judged. For example, she wanted to lose the weight that she had gained since the births of her children (current body mass index [BMI] 27.7) but was afraid of the ridicule that might accompany her efforts at the gym. She had gradually withdrawn from situations in which she might be forced to meet new people, and this made it almost impossible for her to interview for a new job, much less work in one. She had been successfully treated for social phobia 5 years earlier with psychotherapy, a selective serotonin reuptake inhibitor (SSRI) antidepressant, and clonazepam 0.25 mg twice daily, but her symptoms had returned over the prior year. She denied increasing the dose of either medication or taking any other medication (prescribed or over the counter) for anxiety. Although excited about her new relationship, she was worried her new girlfriend would leave her if she did not "tune up my act."

She denied periods of significant depression, although she said she had experienced multiple periods of feeling frustrated with her limited effectiveness. She also denied all manic symptoms.

The psychiatrist then asked Ms. Kleber about her "sleepiness." She said she slept more than anyone she knew. She said she typically slept at least 9 hours per night but then took two naps for 5 additional hours during the day. She did not recall a problem until the end of high school, when she started falling asleep around 8:00 or 9:00 P.M. and dozing every afternoon. When she tried to go to college, she realized how much more sleep she needed than her friends and eventually dropped out because she could not stay awake in class. Despite the naps, she typically fell asleep when visiting friends or family and when reading or watching TV. She quit driving alone for fear of falling asleep at the wheel. Late afternoon naps were not restorative and had no apparent impact on her falling asleep at night.

Raising a family was difficult, especially because mornings were Ms. Kleber's worst period. For at least half an hour after waking, she was disoriented and confused, making it difficult to get her children to school. Throughout the day, she said she felt "scattered and inattentive."

Snoring had appeared 5 years earlier. Her companion was unsure whether Ms. Kleber also had breathing pauses during her sleep. Ms. Kleber denied having ever experienced sleep paralysis or abruptly falling asleep in the middle of a sentence. Although she would fall asleep while socializing, it would generally occur during a lull in the conversation while she was in a quiet spot in the corner of a couch. She denied falling down when she fell asleep. She reported experiencing hypnopompic hallucinations several times per year since she was a teenager.

On examination, Ms. Kleber was an overweight woman who was cooperative and coherent. She was concerned about her anxiety but preoccupied with her sleep problem. She denied depression, suicidality, psychosis, and memory complaints. Her insight and judgment appeared intact.

Her physical examination was essentially noncontributory. Her medical history was significant only for hypercholesterolemia and occasional migraine headaches. Ms. Kleber did have some muscular complaints, such as weakness in her legs and pain in her left arm; these were related to exertion. She has smoked marijuana occasionally to help with her pain but denied that the marijuana was an important contributor to her sleepiness. She denied a history of head trauma and unusual illnesses. She denied a family history of sleep or mood problems, although multiple relatives were "anxious."

Ms. Kleber was referred for sleep studies. Polysomnography showed an apnea hypopnea index of 3 events per hour. The next day, she underwent a multiple sleep latency test (MSLT), which indicated a mean sleep latency of 7 minutes with one sleep-onset REM period during the testing. A lumbar puncture was done to assess cerebrospinal fluid (CSF) levels of hypocretin-1; the level appeared in the normal range.

Diagnoses

- Social phobia
- Hypersomnolence disorder

Discussion

Ms. Kleber appears to have several DSM-5 diagnoses that warrant clinical attention. She has been diagnosed with social phobia in the past, and its recurrence seems to have led to this psychiatric consultation. She has gained weight since the birth of her children, and her obesity exacerbates her social avoidance and puts her at risk for sleep disturbances and medical complications. Obesity is not a diagnosis in the main text of DSM-5, but it is listed in the DSM-5 chapter "Other Conditions That May Be a Focus of Clinical Attention." Ms. Kleber's anxiety and weight issues might both warrant independent clinical attention, but it is her sleep problems that appear to most profoundly affect her life.

Ms. Kleber sleeps too much. The sleep is not restful or restorative. Because of the sleep problems, she can barely function as a mother and she indicates that she cannot keep or maintain a job, drive independently, or socialize with friends. She is worried she will lose her new romantic partner. The excess sleep and sleepiness have apparently occurred daily since she neared the end of high school. Ms. Kleber's symptoms are indicative of DSM-5 hypersomnolence disorder. Criteria include symptoms at least 3 days per week for at least 3 months (Ms. Kleber has had symptoms almost daily for over 15 years). The nocturnal sleep duration (9 hours) alone might not suggest a problem, but her total daily sleep duration of 14 hours is typical of hypersomnolence, as are her inertia upon awakening and her unexpected lapses into sleep.

It is important to rule out other explanations for her somnolence. Ms. Kleber smokes marijuana and uses a benzodiazepine for anxiety. She insists that her use is either occasional (the marijuana) or at a low, stable dose (the clonazepam), and that her symptoms predated her use of either. Although both can be sedating, they do not appear to be causative agents. She has pain and headaches, so it would be useful to tactfully inquire further about her possible use of pain medications, which can be sedating. She also describes demoralization about her lack of effectiveness, which should prompt a consideration of depression, which can lead to excessive amounts of nonrestorative sleep. At the moment, none of these possibilities seems likely.

There are multiple sleep disorders that can lead to excessive sleep and/or daytime somnolence. Ms. Kleber's obesity, excessive sleepiness, and snoring should prompt a consideration of sleep apnea, and a sleep study was certainly indicated. Polysomnography yielded an apnea hypopnea index of 3 events per hour, which is in the normal range and indicates that Ms. Kleber does not have a sleep-related breathing disorder.

Ms. Kleber should also be evaluated for narcolepsy, which is characterized by recurrent periods of an irrepressible need to sleep, lapsing into sleep, or napping within the same day. Ms. Kleber's clinical picture is suggestive. Not only does she fall asleep abruptly, but she has relatively frequent hypnopompic hallucinations. Although generally considered normal, hypnopompic hallucinations can reflect sleep-onset REM intrusions and are, therefore, suggestive of narcolepsy. To satisfy requirements for DSM-5 narcolepsy, the individual should demonstrate cataplexy, CSF hypocretin deficiency, or a reduction of REM sleep latency during nocturnal polysomnography or an MSLT. Ms. Kleber's MSLT showed a mean sleep latency of 7 minutes with only one sleep-onset REM period during the testing. The sleep latency is brief; however, to qualify for narcolepsy, she would need at least two early REM periods during the study. Levels of CSF hypocretin-1 appeared in the normal range, which rules out narcolepsy-cataplexy/hypocretin deficiency syndrome. Unless her episodes of falling asleep are viewed as cataplexy, Ms. Kleber would not qualify for a narcolepsy diagnosis. At this point, then, Ms. Kleber qualifies only for DSM-5 hypersomnolence disorder in addition to her social phobia.

Suggested Readings

Karasu SR, Karasu TB: The Gravity of Weight: A Clinical Guide to Weight Loss and Maintenance. Washington, DC, American Psychiatric Publishing, 2010

Ohayon MM, Reynolds CF 3rd: Epidemiological and clinical relevance of insomnia diagnosis algorithms according to the DSM-IV and the International Classification of Sleep Disorders (ICSD). Sleep Med 10(9):952–960, 2009

Ohayon MM, Dauvilliers Y, Reynolds CF 3rd: Operational definitions and algorithms for excessive sleepiness in the general population: implications for DSM-5 nosology. Arch Gen Psychiatry 69(1):71–79, 2012

Case 3: Sleepiness

Brian Palen, M.D.
Vishesh K. Kapur, M.D., M.P.H.

César Lopez, a 57-year-old Hispanic man, presented for reevaluation of his antidepressant medication. He described several months of worsening fatigue, daytime sleepiness, and generally "not feeling good." He lacked the energy to do his usual activities, but he still enjoyed them when he did participate. He had been having some trouble focusing on his work as an information technology consultant and was worried that he would lose his job. An SSRI antidepressant had been started 2 years earlier, resulting in some improvement of symptoms, and Mr. Lopez insisted he was adherent to this medication.

He denied stressors. In addition to having been diagnosed with depression, he had hypertension, diabetes, and coronary artery disease. He complained of heartburn as well as erectile dysfunction, for which he had not been medically evaluated.

Mr. Lopez was born in Venezuela. He was married and had two grown children. He did not consume tobacco or alcohol but did drink several servings of coffee each day to help maintain alertness.

On physical examination, he was 5 feet 10 inches tall, weighed 235 pounds, and had a BMI of 34. His neck circumference was 20 inches. His respiratory rate was 90, and his blood pressure was 155/90. No other abnormalities were present.

On mental status examination, the patient was a heavyset, cooperative man who appeared tired but was without depressed mood, anxiety, psychosis, or cognitive decline.

More focused questioning revealed that Mr. Lopez not only had trouble staying awake at work, but also occasionally nodded off while driving. He slept 8–10 hours nightly but had frequent awakenings, made nightly trips to the bathroom (nocturia), and often woke with a choking sensation and sometimes with a headache. He had snored since childhood, but he added, "All the men in my family are snorers." Before she elected to sleep nightly in their guest bedroom, his wife said he snored very loudly and intermittently stopped breathing and gasped for air.

Mr. Lopez was sent for a sleep study (polysomnography). Results included the following:

- Apnea hypopnea index: 25 events per hour
- Oxygen desaturation index: 20 events per hour
- Nadir oxygen saturation: 82%
- % Time with oxygen saturation <90%: 8%
- Arousal index: 35 events per hour

- Sleep stage (%):

    % Time in stage N1 sleep: 20%
    % Time in stage N2 sleep: 60%
    % Time in stage N3 sleep: 10%
    % Time in REM sleep: 10%

Diagnosis

- Obstructive sleep apnea hypopnea, moderate severity

Discussion

Mr. Lopez presents for a reevaluation of his treatment for depression, but his presenting symptoms are much more notable for fatigue and sleepiness than for a mood disorder. The patient's history of loud snoring and episodes of choking and gasping suggest that his most likely underlying problem is obstructive sleep apnea hypopnea (OSAH).

Although OSAH affects about 3% of the overall population, rates are much higher in people with pertinent risk factors. Mr. Lopez, for example, is above age 50, is obese with a large neck circumference, and has a family history notable for "all the men" being snorers. Snoring is a particularly sensitive indicator for OSAH, especially when very loud, occurring more than 3 days per week, and accompanied by episodes of choking and gasping. As seen in Mr. Lopez, patients with OSAH also frequently report nocturia, heartburn, sexual dysfunction, and morning headaches, reflecting the multisystem effects of this disorder.

OSAH is characterized by the repetitive collapse (apnea) or partial collapse (hypopnea) of the pharyngeal airway during sleep. Relaxation of the pharyngeal muscles during sleep allows soft tissue in the back of the throat to block the pharyngeal airway. The resultant decrease in airflow can cause significant reductions in blood oxygen saturation. The increased work of breathing through an occluded airway stimulates brief arousals to allow resumption of normal breathing. This pattern can repeat itself hundreds of times throughout the night, resulting in significantly fragmented sleep patterns.

Sleep studies (polysomnography) quantify sleep in multiple ways, but DSM-5 focuses specifically on the apnea hypopnea index (AHI), which is a measure of the number of complete breathing pauses (apneas) and partial breathing events (hypopneas) that last for at least 10 seconds per hour of sleep. If patients have at least 15 obstructive apneas or hypopneas per hour (an AHI of 15), they meet criteria regardless of associated symptoms. With at least five such episodes (an AHI of 5), patients must also have either nocturnal breathing disturbances or daytime sleepiness or fatigue.

The AHI is also the determinant of the severity of OSAH. Mild cases are associated with an AHI of less than 15 (which, by definition, includes some sort of symptoms). Mr. Lopez's 25 events per hour fall in the moderate range of 15–30. OSAH is considered to be severe if the AHI is greater than 30.

Although not specifically related to DSM-5 criteria, Mr. Lopez's polysomnography is notable for abnormal sleep architecture, with a reduction of the percentage of time spent in REM and stage N3 sleep. It demonstrates elevated amounts of time spent with oxygen saturation below 90%, and his arousal index, which measures cortical arousals per hour, is 35, far above the 20 that is the high range of normal.

OSAH is similar to many DSM-5 diagnoses in that if untreated, it can have a seriously negative impact on quality of life. OSAH is unusual within DSM-5, however, in that its diagnosis is heavily based on the results of a test rather than on clinical observation. As exemplified in the case of Mr. Lopez, many people with this disorder do not get promptly diagnosed, leading to extended periods of not receiving adequate treatment. Interestingly, one of the most "objective" of psychiatric diagnoses is only considered during a sensitive clinical assessment.

Suggested Readings

Peppard PE, Szklo-Coxe M, Hla KM, Young T: Longitudinal association of sleep-related breathing disorder and depression. Arch Intern Med 166(16):1709–1715, 2006

Schwartz DJ, Karatinos G: For individuals with obstructive sleep apnea, institution of CPAP therapy is associated with an amelioration of symptoms of depression which is sustained long term. J Clin Sleep Med 15(6):631–635, 2007

Sharafkhaneh A, Giray N, Richardson P, et al: Association of psychiatric disorders and sleep apnea in a large cohort. Sleep 28(11):1405–1411, 2005

Young T, Palta M, Dempsey J, et al: The occurrence of sleep-disordered breathing among middle-aged adults. N Engl J Med 328(17):1230–1235, 1993

Young T, Shahar E, Nieto FJ, et al: Predictors of sleep-disordered breathing in community dwelling adults: the Sleep Heart Health Study. Arch Intern Med 162(8):893–900, 2002

Case 4: Feeling Itchy, Creepy, and Crawly

Kathy P. Parker, Ph.D., R.N.

Dingxiang Meng was a 63-year-old Chinese-born man who was referred for a psychiatric consultation for depression and excessive somatic complaints. He had a history of psychotic depressions for which he had been admitted twice in the prior decade. He was evaluated as an outpatient in the renal unit of a small hospital during his routine hemodialysis.

At the time of the evaluation, Mr. Meng said he felt "itchy, creepy, and crawly," like "worms were crawling underneath the skin." These symptoms had fluctuated over the prior few years but had worsened in recent weeks, and he felt like he was "going crazy." He said he was worried and often tired but said he always laughed when playing with his grandchildren or when visiting with people from his home country. He did not display a thought disorder. A review of the chart indicated that Mr. Meng's physical complaints had been conceptualized at various times as akathisia, peripheral neuropathy, and "psychosomatic" and "psychotically ruminative" symptoms. He had been euthymic and off all psychiatric medications for 2 years at the time of this evaluation.

Mr. Meng said his physical symptoms were worse at night when he tried to sit still or lie down. He said the discomfort was only in his legs. Rubbing them helped, but the greatest relief came from standing up and pacing. Dialysis was especially difficult because of "being strapped to a machine for hours." He also complained of daytime sleepiness and fatigue. In the course of the interview, Mr. Meng twice jumped up from receiving the dialysis. One of the nurses mentioned that he often asked to cut short his dialysis, generally looked tired, and always seemed to be "jumping around."

Mr. Meng had been diagnosed with diabetes soon after his immigration to the United States 15 years earlier. He developed progressive renal insufficiency and had begun hemodialysis 7 years earlier. He was divorced, with two adult children and three young grandchildren. He spoke little English; all interviews were done using a Mandarin interpreter. He lived with one of his children.

Diagnosis

- Restless legs syndrome

Discussion

Mr. Meng presents with depression, fatigue, a creepy sensation of "worms" crawling under his skin, and an intense urge to move. It was not clear to earlier examiners whether his hospitalizations for "psychotic depression" were related to these physical sensations. These sensations were diagnosed in multiple ways over the years: as akathisia, peripheral neuropathy, and "psychosomatic" and "psychotically ruminative" symptoms.

Instead of these diagnoses, Mr. Meng most likely has restless legs syndrome (RLS). A newly independent diagnosis in DSM-5, RLS is characterized by an urge to move the legs, usually accompanied by disagreeable sensations. Mr. Meng's symptoms are typical. The symptoms are improved by movement and are most intense in the evening or when the person is in some sort of sedentary situation (such as dialysis). The symptoms are frequent, chronic, and distressing.

RLS is a particularly common problem for people with end-stage renal disease (ESRD) who are undergoing dialysis. Usually, but not always, the condition is associated with periodic limb movements: stereotypical movements involving extension of the big toe with partial flexing of the ankle, knee, and sometimes hip. Mr. Meng's daytime sleepiness could be related to a delayed sleep onset but also to a reduction in the quality of his sleep; RLS is associated with both problems. ESRD and dialysis are adequate explanations for the RLS (which often has no explanation), but a search should be made for such contributors as anemia, folate deficiency, and uremia. Although obviously not applicable to Mr. Meng, pregnancy is also associated with RLS.

It is not clear why the RLS diagnosis was delayed, especially since RLS is such a common finding in dialysis units. Mr. Meng's history of psychotic depressions might have led the treating team to assume that his complaints were psychological. Such an understanding might have led to the diagnosis of "psychosomatic" symptoms, implying that his physical symptoms were attributable to some sort of psychological disorder or conflict. Not only does that appear to be a misunderstanding of Mr. Meng's complaints, it is a misuse of the term *psychosomatic*, which is better conceptualized as the branch of psychiatry that focuses on comorbidity between psychiatric and medical illnesses; using that definition, it is meaningless to describe someone as "psychoso-matic." Because Mr. Meng was taking antipsychotic medication for at least some of the time that he was also symptomatic, it does make some sense that akathisia was considered. Newer antipsychotic medications (i.e., the atypical antipsychotics) are rarely implicated in akathisia, however, and his symptoms persisted 2 years after the discontinuation of all psychiatric medication. Peripheral neuropathy tends to cause pain, burning, and numbness in the extremities, which is not exactly Mr. Meng's actual complaint.

Perhaps of most concern are the chart notes that indicate that Mr. Meng's restless legs were a manifestation of "psychotic rumination." Communication difficulties may have contributed to this understanding, but it is possible that Mr. Meng's two psychiatric admissions for "psychotic depression" might have actually been precipitated by the somatic preoccupations, anxiety, and dysphoria caused by an undiagnosed case of RLS—a disorder that, although new to DSM-5 as a diagnosis, has long been found to be troublesome and is frequently comorbid with a number of medical illnesses.

Suggested Readings

Araujo SM, de Bruin VM, Nepomuceno LA, et al: Restless legs syndrome in end-stage renal disease: clinical characteristics and associated comorbidities. Sleep Med 11(8):785–790, 2010

Hening W, Allen RP, Tenzer P, Winkelman JW: Restless legs syndrome: demographics, presentation, and differential diagnosis. Geriatrics 62(9):26–29, 2007

La Manna G, Pizza F, Persici E, et al: Restless legs syndrome enhances cardiovascular risk and mortality in patients with end-stage kidney disease undergoing long-term haemodialysis treatment. Nephrol Dial Transplant 26(6):1976–1983, 2011

Li Y, Walters AS, Chiuve SE, et al: Prospective study of restless legs syndrome and coronary heart disease among women. Circulation 126(14):1689–1694, 2012

Oka Y, Ioue Y: Secondary restless legs syndrome [in Japanese]. Brain Nerve 61(5): 539–547, 2009

Winkelman JW, Chertow GM, Lazarus JM: Restless legs syndrome in end-stage renal disease. Am J Kidney Dis 28(3):372–378, 1996

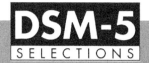

Sleep-Wake Disorders

DSM-5® Self-Exam Questions

1. Which of the following is a core feature of insomnia disorder?

    A. Depressed mood.
    B. Dissatisfaction with sleep quantity or quality.
    C. Cognitive impairment.
    D. Abnormal behaviors during sleep.
    E. Daytime fatigue.

2. Which of the following is necessary to make a diagnosis of insomnia disorder?

    A. Difficulty being fully awake after awakening.
    B. Difficulty with sleep initiation or sleep maintenance, or early-morning awakening with inability to return to sleep.
    C. Absence of a coexisting mental disorder.
    D. Documented insufficient opportunity for sleep.
    E. Persistence of sleep difficulties despite use of sedative-hypnotic agents.

3. An 80-year-old man has a history of myocardial infarction and had coronary artery bypass graft surgery 8 years ago. He plays tennis three times a week, takes care of his grandchildren 2 afternoons each week, generally enjoys life, and manages all of his activities of daily living independently; however, he complains of excessively early morning awakening. He goes to sleep at 9:00 P.M. and sleeps well, with nocturia once nightly, but wakes at 3:30 A.M. although he would like to rise at 5:00 A.M. He does not endorse daytime sleepiness as a problem. His physical examination, mental status, and cognitive function are normal. What is the most likely sleep-wake disorder diagnosis?

    A. Insomnia disorder.
    B. Rapid eye movement (REM) sleep behavior disorder.
    C. Restless legs syndrome.
    D. Obstructive sleep apnea hypopnea.
    E. The man is a short sleeper, which is not a DSM-5 diagnosis.

4. Which of the following symptoms is most likely to indicate the presence of hypersomnolence disorder?

   A. Sleep inertia.
   B. Nonrefreshing sleep in main sleep episode.
   C. Automatic behavior.
   D. Frequent napping.
   E. Headache.

5. An obese 52-year-old man complains of daytime sleepiness, and his partner confirms that he snores, snorts, and gasps during nighttime sleep. What polysomnographic finding is needed to confirm the diagnosis of obstructive sleep apnea hypopnea?

   A. No polysomnography is necessary.
   B. Polysomnographic evidence of at least 5 apnea or hypopnea episodes per hour of sleep.
   C. Polysomnographic evidence of at least 10 apnea or hypopnea episodes per hour of sleep.
   D. Polysomnographic evidence of at least 15 apnea or hypopnea episodes per hour of sleep.
   E. Polysomnographic evidence of resolution of apneas/hypopneas with application of continuous positive airway pressure.

6. In addition to requiring recurrent sleep attacks, the diagnostic criteria for narcolepsy require the presence of cataplexy, hypocretin deficiency, *or* characteristic abnormalities on sleep polysomnography or multiple sleep latency testing. Which of the following is a defining characteristic of cataplexy?

   A. It is sudden.
   B. It is induced by suggestion.
   C. It occurs unilaterally.
   D. It persists for hours.
   E. It is accompanied by hypertonia.

7. In DSM-IV, the diagnosis of breathing-related sleep disorder would be given to an individual complaining of excessive daytime sleepiness, with nocturnal polysomnography demonstrating episodic loss of ventilatory effort and resulting apneic episodes occurring 10–20 times per hour, whose symptoms cannot be attributed to another mental disorder, a medication or substance, or another medical condition. What is the appropriate DSM-5 diagnosis for the same individual?

   A. Insomnia disorder.
   B. Narcolepsy.
   C. Obstructive sleep apnea hypopnea.
   D. Central sleep apnea.
   E. Other specified hypersomnolence disorder.

8. Which of the following metabolic changes is the cardinal feature of sleep-related hypoventilation?

   A. Insulin resistance.
   B. Hypoxia.
   C. Hypercapnia.
   D. Low arterial hemoglobin oxygen saturation.
   E. Elevated vasopressin.

9. A 51-year-old man presents with symptoms of chronic fatigue and excessive worrying about current life stressors. He has a strong family history of depression and a past history of a major depressive episode, with some improvement while maintained on antidepressants. On weekday nights, it takes him several hours to fall asleep, and he then has difficulty getting up to go to work in the morning, experiencing sleepiness for the first few hours of awake time. On weekends, he awakens later in the morning and feels less fatigue and sleepiness. Which of the following diagnoses apply?

   A. Major depressive disorder, in partial remission.
   B. Generalized anxiety disorder.
   C. Insomnia disorder.
   D. Major depressive disorder in partial remission and circadian rhythm sleep-wake disorder, delayed sleep phase type.
   E. Major depressive disorder in partial remission; generalized anxiety disorder; circadian rhythm sleep-wake disorder, delayed sleep phase type; and insomnia disorder.

10. A 67-year-old woman complains of insomnia. She does not have trouble falling asleep between 10 and 11 P.M., but after 1–2 hours she awakens for several hours in the middle of the night, sleeps again for 2–4 hours in the early morning, and then naps three or four times during the day for 1–3 hours at a time. She has a family history of dementia. On exam she appears fatigued and has deficits in short-term memory, calculation, and abstraction. What is the most likely diagnosis?

    A. Major neurocognitive disorder (NCD).
    B. Circadian rhythm sleep-wake disorder, irregular sleep-wake type, and unspecified NCD.
    C. Narcolepsy.
    D. Insomnia disorder.
    E. Major depressive disorder.

11. Following a traumatic brain injury resulting in blindness, a 50-year-old man develops waxing and waning daytime sleepiness interfering with daytime activity. Serial actigraphy (a method of measuring human activity/rest cycles) demonstrates that the time of onset of the major sleep period occurs progres-

sively later day after day, with a normal duration of the major sleep period. What is the most likely diagnosis?

A. Circadian rhythm sleep-wake disorder, unspecified type.
B. Circadian rhythm sleep-wake disorder, delayed sleep phase type.
C. Circadian rhythm sleep-wake disorder, non-24-hour sleep-wake type.
D. Pineal gland injury.
E. Malingering.

12. A 50-year-old emergency department nurse complains of sleepiness at work interfering with her ability to function. She recently switched from the 7 A.M.– 4 P.M. day shift to the 11 P.M.–8 A.M. night shift in order to have her afternoons free. Even with this schedule change, she finds it difficult to sleep in the mornings at home, has little energy for recreational activities or household chores in the afternoon, and feels exhausted by the middle of her overnight shift. What is the most likely diagnosis?

A. Normal variation in sleep secondary to shift work.
B. Circadian rhythm sleep-wake disorder, shift work type.
C. Bipolar disorder.
D. Insomnia disorder.
E. Hypersomnolence disorder.

13. A 14-year-old girl frequently wakes in the morning with clear recollection of very frightening dreams. Once she awakens, she is normally alert and oriented, but the dreams are a persistent source of distress. Her mother reports that the girl sometimes murmurs or groans but does not talk or move during the period before waking. Her history is otherwise notable for having been homeless and living with her mother in a series of temporary shelter accommodations for 1 year when she was 10 years old. What is the most likely diagnosis?

A. Unspecified anxiety disorder.
B. Rapid eye movement (REM) sleep behavior disorder.
C. Non–rapid eye movement sleep arousal disorders.
D. Posttraumatic stress disorder.
E. Nightmare disorder.

14. Which of the following is a type of non–rapid eye movement (REM) sleep arousal disorder in DSM-5?

A. REM sleep behavior disorder.
B. Sleep terrors.
C. Nightmare disorder.
D. Fugue.
E. Obstructive sleep apnea hypopnea.

15. Which of the following is a specific subtype of non–rapid eye movement sleep arousal disorder, sleepwalking type?

    A. Rapid eye movement (REM) sleep behavior disorder.
    B. Sleep-related seizure disorder.
    C. Sleep-related sexual behavior (sexsomnia).
    D. Complex motor behavior during alcoholic blackout.
    E. Nocturnal panic attack.

16. What is the difference between sleep terrors and nightmare disorder?

    A. In nightmare disorder, arousal or awakening from the nightmare is incomplete, whereas sleep terrors result in complete awakening.
    B. In sleep terrors, episodes are concentrated in the final hours of the sleep period, whereas nightmares occur mostly early in the sleep period.
    C. Sleep terrors are characterized by clear recall of vivid dreams with frightening content, whereas nightmares are not recalled.
    D. Sleep terrors occur during rapid eye movement (REM) sleep, whereas nightmares occur in non-REM sleep.
    E. Sleep terrors are precipitous but incomplete awakenings from sleep beginning with a panicky scream or cry, with little recall, whereas nightmares are characterized by full arousal and vivid recall.

17. What is the key abnormality in sleep physiology in rapid eye movement (REM) sleep behavior disorder?

    A. REM starts earlier than normal in the sleep cycle.
    B. There is more REM sleep than normal.
    C. Delta wave activity is increased.
    D. Skeletal muscle tone is preserved during REM sleep.
    E. Total sleep time is greater than normal.

18. Which of the following conditions is commonly associated with rapid eye movement (REM) sleep behavior disorder?

    A. Attention-deficit/hyperactivity disorder.
    B. Synucleinopathies.
    C. Tourette's syndrome.
    D. Sleep terrors.
    E. Epilepsy.

19. Which of the following classes of psychotropic drugs may result in rapid eye movement (REM) sleep without atonia and REM sleep behavior disorder?

   A. Selective serotonin reuptake inhibitors.
   B. Benzodiazepines.
   C. Phenothiazines.
   D. Second-generation antipsychotics.
   E. Monoamine oxidase inhibitors.

20. A 10-year-old boy is referred by his teacher for evaluation of his difficulty sitting still in school, which is interfering with his academic performance. The boy complains of an unpleasant "creepy-crawly" sensation in his legs and an urge to move them when sitting still that is relieved by movement. This symptom bothers him most of the day, but less when playing sports after school or watching television in the evening, and it generally does not bother him in bed at night. What aspect of his clinical presentation rules out a diagnosis of restless legs syndrome (RLS)?

   A. He is too young for a diagnosis of RLS.
   B. He does not have a sleep complaint.
   C. He does not complain of daytime fatigue or sleepiness.
   D. His symptoms occur in the daytime as much as or more than in the evening or at night.
   E. He does not have impaired social functioning.

21. A 28-year-old woman who is in her thirty-fourth week of pregnancy reports that for the past few weeks she has experienced restlessness and difficulty falling asleep at the onset of the sleep period, as well as daytime fatigue. She works during the day and has not changed her schedule. She states that as she becomes increasingly tired, she feels more irritable and depressed. What sleep disorder is suggested by the onset of these symptoms in the third trimester of pregnancy?

   A. Circadian rhythm sleep-wake disorder, delayed sleep phase type.
   B. Insomnia disorder.
   C. Rapid eye movement (REM) sleep behavior disorder.
   D. Restless legs syndrome.
   E. Hypersomnolence disorder.

22. Which of the following sleep disturbances or disorders occurs during rapid eye movement (REM) sleep?

   A. Nightmare disorder.
   B. Confusional arousals.
   C. Sleep terrors.
   D. Obstructive sleep apnea hypopnea.
   E. Central sleep apnea.

23. Which of the following sleep disturbances is associated with chronic opiate use?

    A. Excessive daytime sleepiness.
    B. Insomnia.
    C. Periodic limb movements in sleep.
    D. Obstructive sleep apnea hypopnea.
    E. Parasomnias.

24. Which of the following substances is associated with parasomnias?

    A. Cannabis.
    B. Zolpidem.
    C. Methadone.
    D. Cocaine.
    E. Mescaline.

25. A psychiatric consultation is requested for evaluation and help with management of severe insomnia in a 65-year-old man, beginning the day after elective hip replacement surgery and continuing for 2 days. On evaluation the patient acknowledges heavy drinking until the day before surgery, and he appears to be in alcohol withdrawal, with autonomic instability, confusion, and tremor. Why would a diagnosis of substance/medication-induced sleep disorder be inappropriate in this situation?

    A. The insomnia is an understandable emotional reaction to the anxiety provoked by having surgery.
    B. The insomnia is not causing functional impairment.
    C. The insomnia has not been documented with polysomnography or actigraphy.
    D. The insomnia is occurring during acute alcohol withdrawal.
    E. The insomnia might be related to postoperative pain.

26. A 56-year-old college professor complains of having difficulty sleeping for more than 5 hours per night over the past few weeks, leaving her feeling tired in the daytime. She awakens an hour or two before her intended waking time in the morning, experiencing restless sleep with frequent awakenings until it is time to get up. She does not have initial insomnia and is not depressed. The patient attributes the sleep trouble to intrusive thoughts that arise, after she initially awakens momentarily, about the need to complete an overdue academic project. What is the most appropriate diagnosis?

    A. Adjustment disorder with anxious mood.
    B. Obsessive-compulsive personality disorder.
    C. Insomnia disorder.
    D. Other specified insomnia disorder (brief insomnia disorder).
    E. Unspecified insomnia disorder.

27. A 74-year-old woman has a history of daytime sleepiness interfering with her ability to carry out her daily routine. She reports that it has become progressively worse over the past year. Polysomnography reveals sleep apnea without evidence of airway obstruction with two or three apneic episodes per hour. What is the most appropriate diagnosis?

    A. Central sleep apnea.
    B. Other specified sleep-wake disorder (atypical central sleep apnea).
    C. Unspecified sleep-wake disorder.
    D. Rapid eye movement (REM) sleep behavior disorder.
    E. Circadian rhythm sleep-wake disorder.

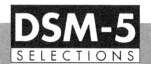

Sleep-Wake Disorders
DSM-5® Self-Exam Answer Guide

1. Which of the following is a core feature of insomnia disorder?

   A. Depressed mood.
   B. Dissatisfaction with sleep quantity or quality.
   C. Cognitive impairment.
   D. Abnormal behaviors during sleep.
   E. Daytime fatigue.

   Correct Answer: B. Dissatisfaction with sleep quantity or quality.

   Explanation: Individuals with insomnia disorder typically present with sleep-wake complaints of dissatisfaction regarding the quality, timing, or amount of sleep. Resulting distress and impairment are core features.

   Insomnia Disorder / diagnostic criteria (p. 362)

2. Which of the following is necessary to make a diagnosis of insomnia disorder?

   A. Difficulty being fully awake after awakening.
   B. Difficulty with sleep initiation or sleep maintenance, or early-morning awakening with inability to return to sleep.
   C. Absence of a coexisting mental disorder.
   D. Documented insufficient opportunity for sleep.
   E. Persistence of sleep difficulties despite use of sedative-hypnotic agents.

   Correct Answer: B. Difficulty with sleep initiation or sleep maintenance, or early-morning awakening with inability to return to sleep.

   Explanation: The key features of insomnia disorder in DSM-5 are dissatisfaction with sleep quality, trouble initiating or maintaining sleep, or early-morning awakening or, in children, resistance to going to bed, and distress or impairment in daytime functioning, despite adequate opportunity to sleep, with the problem occurring frequently and persisting for at least 3 months. An important change from DSM-IV is the possibility of making an independent diagnosis of insomnia disorder even when another disorder such as major depressive disorder might include sleep disturbance as a diagnostic feature. In such a case,

131

both diagnoses would be appropriate, and the comorbid psychiatric disorder listed as a clinical comorbid condition specifier (i.e., "With non–sleep disorder mental comorbidity").

Insomnia Disorder / diagnostic criteria (pp. 362–363)

3. An 80-year-old man has a history of myocardial infarction and had coronary artery bypass graft surgery 8 years ago. He plays tennis three times a week, takes care of his grandchildren 2 afternoons each week, generally enjoys life, and manages all of his activities of daily living independently; however, he complains of excessively early morning awakening. He goes to sleep at 9:00 P.M. and sleeps well, with nocturia once nightly, but wakes at 3:30 A.M. although he would like to rise at 5:00 A.M. He does not endorse daytime sleepiness as a problem. His physical examination, mental status, and cognitive function are normal. What is the most likely sleep-wake disorder diagnosis?

    A. Insomnia disorder.
    B. Rapid eye movement (REM) sleep behavior disorder.
    C. Restless legs syndrome.
    D. Obstructive sleep apnea hypopnea.
    E. The man is a short sleeper, which is not a DSM-5 diagnosis.

Correct Answer: E. The man is a short sleeper, which is not a DSM-5 diagnosis.

Explanation: Although he complains about his sleep timing and endorses early awakening as a complaint, this man has no other features of impairment to justify a diagnosis of insomnia disorder. Many older adults are short sleepers. This man has no evidence of functional impairment such as excessive daytime sleepiness interfering with activities.

Insomnia Disorder / Differential Diagnosis (p. 367)

4. Which of the following symptoms is most likely to indicate the presence of hypersomnolence disorder?

    A. Sleep inertia.
    B. Nonrefreshing sleep in main sleep episode.
    C. Automatic behavior.
    D. Frequent napping.
    E. Headache.

Correct Answer: A. Sleep inertia.

Explanation: Sleep inertia is a period of impaired performance and reduced vigilance, following waking from the main episode of sleep or from a nap that persists for several minutes or more. Although some patients with hypersomnolence disorder have one or more of the other symptoms listed, these symptoms are not as specific to hypersomnolence disorder as is sleep inertia.

Hypersomnolence Disorder / diagnostic criteria; Diagnostic Features (pp. 368–369)

5. An obese 52-year-old man complains of daytime sleepiness, and his partner confirms that he snores, snorts, and gasps during nighttime sleep. What polysomnographic finding is needed to confirm the diagnosis of obstructive sleep apnea hypopnea?

   A. No polysomnography is necessary.
   B. Polysomnographic evidence of at least 5 apnea or hypopnea episodes per hour of sleep.
   C. Polysomnographic evidence of at least 10 apnea or hypopnea episodes per hour of sleep.
   D. Polysomnographic evidence of at least 15 apnea or hypopnea episodes per hour of sleep.
   E. Polysomnographic evidence of resolution of apneas/hypopneas with application of continuous positive airway pressure.

Correct Answer: B. Polysomnographic evidence of at least 5 apnea or hypopnea episodes per hour of sleep.

Explanation: The diagnostic criteria for obstructive sleep apnea hypopnea are as follows:

A. Either (1) or (2):

   1. Evidence by polysomnography of at least five obstructive apneas or hypopneas per hour of sleep and either of the following sleep symptoms:

      a. Nocturnal breathing disturbances: snoring, snorting/gasping, or breathing pauses during sleep.
      b. Daytime sleepiness, fatigue, or unrefreshing sleep despite sufficient opportunities to sleep that is not better explained by another mental disorder (including a sleep disorder) and is not attributable to another medical condition.

   2. Evidence by polysomnography of 15 or more obstructive apneas and/or hypopneas per hour of sleep regardless of accompanying symptoms.

Obstructive Sleep Apnea Hypopnea / diagnostic criteria (p. 378)

6. In addition to requiring recurrent sleep attacks, the diagnostic criteria for narcolepsy require the presence of cataplexy, hypocretin deficiency, *or* characteristic abnormalities on sleep polysomnography or multiple sleep latency testing. Which of the following is a defining characteristic of cataplexy?

   A. It is sudden.
   B. It is induced by suggestion.

C. It occurs unilaterally.
D. It persists for hours.
E. It is accompanied by hypertonia.

Correct Answer: A. It is sudden.

Explanation: The definition of cataplexy differs according to patient character-istics. In individuals with long-standing narcolepsy, cataplexy is defined as brief (seconds to minutes) episodes of sudden bilateral loss of muscle tone with maintained consciousness that are precipitated by laughter or joking. In children or in individuals within 6 months of onset, cataplexy takes the form of spontane-ous grimaces or jaw-opening episodes with tongue thrusting or a global hypo-tonia, without any obvious emotional triggers.

Narcolepsy / diagnostic criteria (pp. 372–373)

7. In DSM-IV, the diagnosis of breathing-related sleep disorder would be given to an individual complaining of excessive daytime sleepiness, with nocturnal polysomnography demonstrating episodic loss of ventilatory effort and result-ing apneic episodes occurring 10–20 times per hour, whose symptoms cannot be attributed to another mental disorder, a medication or substance, or another medical condition. What is the appropriate DSM-5 diagnosis for the same in-dividual?

    A. Insomnia disorder.
    B. Narcolepsy.
    C. Obstructive sleep apnea hypopnea.
    D. Central sleep apnea.
    E. Other specified hypersomnolence disorder.

Correct Answer: D. Central sleep apnea.

Explanation: The diagnosis of central sleep apnea is made on the basis of five or more central apneic episodes per hour on polysomnography and absence of another sleep disorder. Unlike DSM-IV, DSM-5 codes central and obstructive sleep apnea syndromes as different diagnoses within a larger group of breath-ing-related sleep disorders that also includes sleep-related hypoventilation. Central apneas are characterized by a loss of respiratory drive rather than by mechanical obstruction.

Central Sleep Apnea / Diagnostic Features (pp. 383–384)

8. Which of the following metabolic changes is the cardinal feature of sleep-related hypoventilation?

    A. Insulin resistance.
    B. Hypoxia.

    C. Hypercapnia.
    D. Low arterial hemoglobin oxygen saturation.
    E. Elevated vasopressin.

Correct Answer: C. Hypercapnia.

Explanation: Sleep-related hypoventilation is diagnosed using polysomnography showing sleep-related hypoxemia and hypercapnia that is not better explained by another breathing-related sleep disorder. The documentation of increased arterial pCO_2 levels to greater than 55 mmHg during sleep or a 10 mmHg or greater increase in pCO_2 levels (to a level that also exceeds 50 mmHg) during sleep in comparison to awake supine values, for 10 minutes or longer, is the gold standard for diagnosis. However, obtaining arterial blood gas determinations during sleep is impractical, and noninvasive measures of pCO_2 have not been adequately validated during sleep and are not widely used during polysomnography in adults. Prolonged and sustained decreases in oxygen saturation (oxygen saturation of less than 90% for more than 5 minutes with a nadir of at least 85%, or oxygen saturation of less than 90% for at least 30% of sleep time) in the absence of evidence of upper airway obstruction are often used as an indication of sleep-related hypoventilation; however, this finding is not specific, as there are other potential causes of hypoxemia, such as that due to lung disease.

Sleep-Related Hypoventilation / Diagnostic Markers (p. 389)

9. A 51-year-old man presents with symptoms of chronic fatigue and excessive worrying about current life stressors. He has a strong family history of depression and a past history of a major depressive episode, with some improvement while maintained on antidepressants. On weekday nights, it takes him several hours to fall asleep, and he then has difficulty getting up to go to work in the morning, experiencing sleepiness for the first few hours of awake time. On weekends, he awakens later in the morning and feels less fatigue and sleepiness. Which of the following diagnoses apply?

    A. Major depressive disorder, in partial remission.
    B. Generalized anxiety disorder.
    C. Insomnia disorder.
    D. Major depressive disorder in partial remission and circadian rhythm sleep-wake disorder, delayed sleep phase type.
    E. Major depressive disorder in partial remission; generalized anxiety disorder; circadian rhythm sleep-wake disorder, delayed sleep phase type; and insomnia disorder.

Correct Answer: D. Major depressive disorder in partial remission and circadian rhythm sleep-wake disorder, delayed sleep phase type.

Explanation: In this case, both diagnoses should be coded, even though insomnia can be considered as a symptom of major depressive disorder. Circadian rhythm sleep-wake disorder, delayed sleep phase type, is characterized by delayed onset (usually more than 2 hours) of the major sleep period in relation to the desired sleep and wake times appropriate to the individual's personal and occupational obligations, with resulting symptoms of tiredness and insomnia complaints. When allowed to set their own schedule, individuals with this condition have normal (for age) quality and quantity of sleep.

Circadian Rhythm Sleep-Wake Disorders / diagnostic criteria (pp. 390–391)

10. A 67-year-old woman complains of insomnia. She does not have trouble falling asleep between 10 and 11 P.M., but after 1–2 hours she awakens for several hours in the middle of the night, sleeps again for 2–4 hours in the early morning, and then naps three or four times during the day for 1–3 hours at a time. She has a family history of dementia. On exam she appears fatigued and has deficits in short-term memory, calculation, and abstraction. What is the most likely diagnosis?

    A. Major neurocognitive disorder (NCD).
    B. Circadian rhythm sleep-wake disorder, irregular sleep-wake type, and unspecified NCD.
    C. Narcolepsy.
    D. Insomnia disorder.
    E. Major depressive disorder.

Correct Answer: B. Circadian rhythm sleep-wake disorder, irregular sleep-wake type, and unspecified NCD.

Explanation: The DSM-5 circadian rhythm sleep-wake disorders retained three of the DSM-IV subtypes—delayed sleep phase type, shift work type, and unspecified type—and expanded to include advanced sleep phase type and irregular sleep-wake type, whereas the jet lag type was removed. In this patient's presentation, there is no major sleep period and no discernible circadian rhythm to the sleep-wake cycle; her sleep is fragmented into five or six periods across the 24-hour day. *Irregular sleep-wake type* is commonly associated with NCDs, including major NCDs such as Alzheimer's disease, Parkinson's disease, and Huntington's disease, as well as NCDs in children. Insufficient data are provided to justify a diagnosis of major NCD or depression. This woman does not have narcolepsy, which is characterized by frequent irresistible urges to sleep, but also requires the presence of at least one of the following: 1) cataplexy, 2) hypocretin deficiency, or 3) characteristic abnormalities on nocturnal polysomnography or multiple sleep latency testing.

Circadian Rhythm Sleep-Wake Disorders / Irregular Sleep-Wake Type (pp. 394–395); Narcolepsy / diagnostic criteria (pp. 372–373)

11. Following a traumatic brain injury resulting in blindness, a 50-year-old man develops waxing and waning daytime sleepiness interfering with daytime activity. Serial actigraphy (a method of measuring human activity/rest cycles) demonstrates that the time of onset of the major sleep period occurs progressively later day after day, with a normal duration of the major sleep period. What is the most likely diagnosis?

    A. Circadian rhythm sleep-wake disorder, unspecified type.
    B. Circadian rhythm sleep-wake disorder, delayed sleep phase type.
    C. Circadian rhythm sleep-wake disorder, non-24-hour sleep-wake type.
    D. Pineal gland injury.
    E. Malingering.

    Correct Answer: C. Circadian rhythm sleep-wake disorder, non-24-hour sleep-wake type.

    Explanation: Non-24-hour sleep-wake type circadian rhythm sleep disorder is common in individuals with blindness. The endogenous sleep-wake cycle is longer than 24 hours and is not entrained by light cues, resulting in onset of sleepiness at later and later times of day. When the onset of sleepiness occurs at night, there is low interference with normal daytime activities; however, as the onset of sleepiness cycles toward the daytime hours there is greater impairment in social-occupational function. In DSM-IV, this disorder was included in the "unspecified" type of circadian rhythm sleep disorder.

    Circadian Rhythm Sleep-Wake Disorders / Diagnostic Features (p. 396)

12. A 50-year-old emergency department nurse complains of sleepiness at work interfering with her ability to function. She recently switched from the 7 A.M.–4 P.M. day shift to the 11 P.M.–8 A.M. night shift in order to have her afternoons free. Even with this schedule change, she finds it difficult to sleep in the mornings at home, has little energy for recreational activities or household chores in the afternoon, and feels exhausted by the middle of her overnight shift. What is the most likely diagnosis?

    A. Normal variation in sleep secondary to shift work.
    B. Circadian rhythm sleep-wake disorder, shift work type.
    C. Bipolar disorder.
    D. Insomnia disorder.
    E. Hypersomnolence disorder.

    Correct Answer: B. Circadian rhythm sleep-wake disorder, shift work type.

    Explanation: The criteria for circadian rhythm sleep-wake disorder, shift work type, are a gradual reversion from conventional daylight hours as the main period of occupational engagement, difficulty sleeping in the day, and sleepiness at night during the work shift. The daylight sleeping problem might be mis-

taken for insomnia and the work shift sleepiness problem for hypersomnolence, but the presence of both symptoms in this context clarifies the diagnosis.
The daytime and nighttime symptoms must be clinically significant in terms of
distress or impairment in function, which is largely a clinical judgment, and the
boundary between normal variation in sleep and sleepiness due to shift work versus the shift work type of circadian rhythm sleep-wake disorder is not sharply
demarcated. Bipolar disorder may be destabilized by shift work that interferes
with stable circadian rhythms and adequate sleep at nighttime, but mania resulting from such destabilization does not generally manifest as complaints of
sleepiness or insomnia.

Circadian Rhythm Sleep-Wake Disorders / Shift Work Type (pp. 397–398)

13. A 14-year-old girl frequently wakes in the morning with clear recollection of
very frightening dreams. Once she awakens, she is normally alert and oriented, but the dreams are a persistent source of distress. Her mother reports
that the girl sometimes murmurs or groans but does not talk or move during
the period before waking. Her history is otherwise notable for having been
homeless and living with her mother in a series of temporary shelter accommodations for 1 year when she was 10 years old. What is the most likely diagnosis?

    A. Unspecified anxiety disorder.
    B. Rapid eye movement (REM) sleep behavior disorder.
    C. Non–rapid eye movement sleep arousal disorders.
    D. Posttraumatic stress disorder.
    E. Nightmare disorder.

Correct Answer: E. Nightmare disorder.

Explanation: Nightmare disorder is characterized by repeated nightmares,
which are extended, dysphoric, and well-remembered dreams occurring mostly
in the second half of the major sleep episode and which usually involve threats
to one's survival, security, or physical integrity. On awakening, the affected individual returns quickly to a normal level of consciousness with normal orien-
tation, but the dreams cause persistent distress and/or impairment in function.
Coexisting medical and mental disorders do not adequately explain the predominant complaint of dysphoric dreams. In children, nightmare disorder occurs most often after exposure to severe psychosocial stressors. Nightmares
occur during REM sleep, when skeletal muscle tone decreases, so vocalization
and body movement does not occur, except possibly at the very end of the
REM sleep period. Nightmare disorder is common in childhood, and may continue to occur in women into adulthood, but is less common in men in adulthood. In contrast to nightmares, sleep terrors are associated with non-REM deep-
stage sleep, generally occur earlier in the major sleep period, and are characterized by poor recall, only partial arousal, and confusion and disorientation at

the end of the terror event. Amnesia for the event is common after the end of the sleep period. REM sleep behavior disorder is characterized by violent dream enactment or other complex motor behavior during sleep, and it is most common in middle-aged or older, male patients. Nightmares can occur in posttraumatic stress disorder (PTSD) as part of the "reexperiencing" phenomena but are insufficient alone to make a diagnosis of PTSD.

Non–Rapid Eye Movement Sleep Arousal Disorders / diagnostic criteria (p. 399); Nightmare Disorder / diagnostic criteria (p. 404); Rapid Eye Movement Sleep Behavior Disorder / diagnostic criteria (pp. 407–408)

14. Which of the following is a type of non–rapid eye movement (REM) sleep arousal disorder in DSM-5?

    A. REM sleep behavior disorder.
    B. Sleep terrors.
    C. Nightmare disorder.
    D. Fugue.
    E. Obstructive sleep apnea hypopnea.

Correct Answer: B. Sleep terrors.

Explanation: DSM-5 includes sleep terrors and sleepwalking in the diagnostic category of non-REM sleep arousal disorders. *Sleep terrors* are associated with a sense of terror and distress, but with incomplete awakening and poor recall, and they tend to occur early in the major sleep period, when non-REM sleep predominates. *REM sleep behavior disorder* episodes occur in REM sleep, which is predominantly in the later part of the sleep episode, with complex behaviors that are often recalled as "acting out" of a dream, sometimes violently. Nightmares are also a REM sleep phenomenon. Patients with *nightmare disorder* awaken and rapidly reorient and achieve full alertness, in contrast to those with sleep terrors. *Fugue* states are not sleep disorders.

Non–Rapid Eye Movement Sleep Arousal Disorders / diagnostic criteria (p. 399)

15. Which of the following is a specific subtype of non–rapid eye movement sleep arousal disorder, sleepwalking type?

    A. Rapid eye movement (REM) sleep behavior disorder.
    B. Sleep-related seizure disorder.
    C. Sleep-related sexual behavior (sexsomnia).
    D. Complex motor behavior during alcoholic blackout.
    E. Nocturnal panic attack.

Correct Answer: C. Sleep-related sexual behavior (sexsomnia).

Explanation: The essential feature of sleepwalking is repeated episodes of complex motor behavior initiated during sleep, including rising from bed and walking about. Sleep-related sexual behavior and sleep-related eating are recognized as specific subtypes. Sleepwalking arises in non-REM sleep, not during REM sleep. Sleepwalking episodes can begin with a confusional arousal but progress to more complex motor behaviors and ambulation. Alcoholic blackouts do not occur during sleep or unconsciousness but involve loss of memory for events during the drinking episode. Sleep-related seizures are in the differential diagnosis of non-REM sleep arousal disorders but tend to be more stereotypic rather than complex motor behaviors.

Non–Rapid Eye Movement Sleep Arousal Disorders / diagnostic criteria; Diagnostic Features (pp. 399–400)

16. What is the difference between sleep terrors and nightmare disorder?

    A. In nightmare disorder, arousal or awakening from the nightmare is incomplete, whereas sleep terrors result in complete awakening.
    B. In sleep terrors, episodes are concentrated in the final hours of the sleep period, whereas nightmares occur mostly early in the sleep period.
    C. Sleep terrors are characterized by clear recall of vivid dreams with frightening content, whereas nightmares are not recalled.
    D. Sleep terrors occur during rapid eye movement (REM) sleep, whereas nightmares occur in non-REM sleep.
    E. Sleep terrors are precipitous but incomplete awakenings from sleep beginning with a panicky scream or cry, with little recall, whereas nightmares are characterized by full arousal and vivid recall.

Correct Answer: E. Sleep terrors are precipitous but incomplete awakenings from sleep beginning with a panicky scream or cry, with little recall, whereas nightmares are characterized by full arousal and vivid recall.

Explanation: Sleep terrors are a non-REM sleep phenomenon and therefore tend to occur in the early period of sleep when non-REM sleep predominates; autonomic arousal, fearful crying out, incomplete awakening, and little recall or total amnesia characterize the episodes. Nightmares are REM sleep phenomena and therefore tend to be more prominent in the later part of the sleep period, and may be vividly recalled. Arousal after a nightmare tends to be to full consciousness.

Nightmare Disorder / diagnostic criteria (p. 404)

17. What is the key abnormality in sleep physiology in rapid eye movement (REM) sleep behavior disorder?

    A. REM starts earlier than normal in the sleep cycle.
    B. There is more REM sleep than normal.

C. Delta wave activity is increased.

D. Skeletal muscle tone is preserved during REM sleep.

E. Total sleep time is greater than normal.

Correct Answer: D. Skeletal muscle tone is preserved during REM sleep.

Explanation: REM sleep without atonia is a sine qua non for the diagnosis of REM sleep behavior disorder. Normally there is loss of muscle tone during REM sleep, so no voluntary motor activity occurs, but when muscle atonia is not present, the dreaming individual "enacts" his or her actions in the ongoing dream. In an individual with an established synucleinopathy diagnosis, a history suggestive of REM sleep behavior disorder, even in the absence of polysomnographic evidence of REM sleep without atonia, is adequate to make the diagnosis of REM sleep behavior disorder.

Rapid Eye Movement Sleep Behavior Disorder / Diagnostic Features (p. 408)

18. Which of the following conditions is commonly associated with rapid eye movement (REM) sleep behavior disorder?

A. Attention-deficit/hyperactivity disorder.

B. Synucleinopathies.

C. Tourette's syndrome.

D. Sleep terrors.

E. Epilepsy.

Correct Answer: B. Synucleinopathies.

Explanation: Based on findings from individuals presenting to sleep clinics, most individuals (>50%) with initially "idiopathic" REM sleep behavior disorder will eventually develop a neurodegenerative disease—most notably, one of the synucleinopathies (Parkinson's disease, multiple system atrophy, or major or mild neurocognitive disorder with Lewy bodies). REM sleep behavior disorder often predates any other sign of these disorders by many years (often more than a decade). Nocturnal seizures may perfectly mimic REM sleep behavior disorder, but the behaviors are generally more stereotyped. Polysomnographic monitoring employing a full electroencephalographic seizure montage may differentiate the two. REM sleep without atonia is not present on polysomnographic monitoring.

Rapid Eye Movement Sleep Behavior Disorder / Development and Course (p. 408–409)

19. Which of the following classes of psychotropic drugs may result in rapid eye movement (REM) sleep without atonia and REM sleep behavior disorder?

    A. Selective serotonin reuptake inhibitors.
    B. Benzodiazepines.
    C. Phenothiazines.
    D. Second-generation antipsychotics.
    E. Monoamine oxidase inhibitors.

    Correct Answer: A. Selective serotonin reuptake inhibitors.

    Explanation: Many widely prescribed medications, including tricyclic antidepressants, selective serotonin reuptake inhibitors, serotonin-norepinephrine reuptake inhibitors, and beta-blockers, may result in polysomnographic evidence of REM sleep without atonia and in frank REM sleep behavior disorder. It is not known whether the medications per se result in REM sleep behavior disorder or they unmask an underlying predisposition

    Rapid Eye Movement Sleep Behavior Disorder / Risk and Prognostic Factors (p. 409)

20. A 10-year-old boy is referred by his teacher for evaluation of his difficulty sitting still in school, which is interfering with his academic performance. The boy complains of an unpleasant "creepy-crawly" sensation in his legs and an urge to move them when sitting still that is relieved by movement. This symptom bothers him most of the day, but less when playing sports after school or watching television in the evening, and it generally does not bother him in bed at night. What aspect of his clinical presentation rules out a diagnosis of restless legs syndrome (RLS)?

    A. He is too young for a diagnosis of RLS.
    B. He does not have a sleep complaint.
    C. He does not complain of daytime fatigue or sleepiness.
    D. His symptoms occur in the daytime as much as or more than in the evening or at night.
    E. He does not have impaired social functioning.

    Correct Answer: D. His symptoms occur in the daytime as much as or more than in the evening or at night.

    Explanation: The diagnostic criteria for RLS specify that symptoms are worse in the evening or night, and in some individuals occur only in the evening or night. The symptoms can delay sleep onset and awaken the individual from sleep, resulting in significant sleep fragmentation and daytime sleepiness. RLS symptoms are accompanied by significant distress or impairment in social, occupational, educational, academic, behavioral, or other important areas of functioning. Although it is more common in adults, RLS can be diagnosed in children.

Restless Legs Syndrome / diagnostic criteria (p. 410); Diagnostic Features; Development and Course (p. 411)

21. A 28-year-old woman who is in her thirty-fourth week of pregnancy reports that for the past few weeks she has experienced restlessness and difficulty falling asleep at the onset of the sleep period, as well as daytime fatigue. She works during the day and has not changed her schedule. She states that as she becomes increasingly tired, she feels more irritable and depressed. What sleep disorder is suggested by the onset of these symptoms in the third trimester of pregnancy?

    A. Circadian rhythm sleep-wake disorder, delayed sleep phase type.
    B. Insomnia disorder.
    C. Rapid eye movement (REM) sleep behavior disorder.
    D. Restless legs syndrome.
    E. Hypersomnolence disorder.

    Correct Answer: D. Restless legs syndrome.

    Explanation: The onset of symptoms late in pregnancy is a common feature of restless legs syndrome; the prevalence of restless legs syndrome in pregnant women is two to three times higher than that in the general population. In this case, one would want to know more about the patient's sense of restlessness in order to determine whether she has the unpleasant sensations and urge to move her legs, with relief of the unpleasant sensations after moving, that are the hallmark of the disorder.

    Restless Legs Syndrome / Gender-Related Diagnostic Issues (p. 412)

22. Which of the following sleep disturbances or disorders occurs during rapid eye movement (REM) sleep?

    A. Nightmare disorder.
    B. Confusional arousals.
    C. Sleep terrors.
    D. Obstructive sleep apnea hypopnea.
    E. Central sleep apnea.

    Correct Answer: A. Nightmare disorder.

    Explanation: Nightmares occur during REM sleep, which makes up a larger part of the sleep cycle later in the sleep period. Confusional arousals and sleep terrors are non-REM sleep phenomena. Obstructive sleep apneas and especially central sleep apneas tend to occur in deeper stages of sleep but can occur in lighter sleep as well, and they are not REM related.

    Nightmare Disorder / Diagnostic Features (pp. 404–405)

23. Which of the following sleep disturbances is associated with chronic opiate use?

    A. Excessive daytime sleepiness.
    B. Insomnia.
    C. Periodic limb movements in sleep.
    D. Obstructive sleep apnea hypopnea.
    E. Parasomnias.

Correct Answer: B. Insomnia.

Explanation: Although acute opiate intoxication tends to lead to sedation, habituation may result in eventual complaints of insomnia. Opiates may also decrease respiratory drive, resulting in central sleep apneas.

Substance/Medication-Induced Sleep Disorder / Associated Features Supporting Diagnosis (p. 417)

24. Which of the following substances is associated with parasomnias?

    A. Cannabis.
    B. Zolpidem.
    C. Methadone.
    D. Cocaine.
    E. Mescaline.

Correct Answer: B. Zolpidem.

Explanation: Benzodiazepine receptor agonists, especially at high doses, may cause parasomnias. These would be classified as a zolpidem-induced sleep disorder, with onset during intoxication, parasomnia type.

Substance/Medication-Induced Sleep Disorder / Associated Features Supporting Diagnosis (p. 417)

25. A psychiatric consultation is requested for evaluation and help with management of severe insomnia in a 65-year-old man, beginning the day after elective hip replacement surgery and continuing for 2 days. On evaluation the patient acknowledges heavy drinking until the day before surgery, and he appears to be in alcohol withdrawal, with autonomic instability, confusion, and tremor. Why would a diagnosis of substance/medication-induced sleep disorder be inappropriate in this situation?

    A. The insomnia is an understandable emotional reaction to the anxiety provoked by having surgery.
    B. The insomnia is not causing functional impairment.
    C. The insomnia has not been documented with polysomnography or actigraphy.

D. The insomnia is occurring during acute alcohol withdrawal.

E. The insomnia might be related to postoperative pain.

Correct Answer: D. The insomnia is occurring during acute alcohol withdrawal.

Explanation: A substance/medication-induced sleep disorder diagnosis should be made instead of a diagnosis of substance withdrawal only when the sleep disturbance symptoms "predominate in the clinical picture" and are "sufficiently severe to warrant clinical attention." Otherwise, a diagnosis of substance withdrawal is more appropriate. Pain and emotional stress may result in insomnia and should certainly be considered in the differential diagnosis of this patient's problems. Functional impairment may be hard to judge in a medically hospitalized patient, but it can sometimes be understood in terms of the patient's ability to participate appropriately with care. Polysomnography and actigraphy are useful tools in sleep disorder diagnosis in general, but they are not required to make this particular diagnosis.

Substance/Medication-Induced Sleep Disorder / diagnostic criteria (pp. 413–414)

26. A 56-year-old college professor complains of having difficulty sleeping for more than 5 hours per night over the past few weeks, leaving her feeling tired in the daytime. She awakens an hour or two before her intended waking time in the morning, experiencing restless sleep with frequent awakenings until it is time to get up. She does not have initial insomnia and is not depressed. The patient attributes the sleep trouble to intrusive thoughts that arise, after she initially awakens momentarily, about the need to complete an overdue academic project. What is the most appropriate diagnosis?

A. Adjustment disorder with anxious mood.

B. Obsessive-compulsive personality disorder.

C. Insomnia disorder.

D. Other specified insomnia disorder (brief insomnia disorder).

E. Unspecified insomnia disorder.

Correct Answer: D. Other specified insomnia disorder (brief insomnia disorder).

Explanation: According to DSM-5, "The other specified insomnia disorder category is used in situations in which the clinician chooses to communicate the specific reason that the presentation does not meet the criteria for insomnia disorder or any specific sleep-wake disorder. This is done by recording 'other specified insomnia disorder' followed by the specific reason (e.g., brief insomnia disorder)." In this case we do not have sufficient evidence to justify a diagnosis of adjustment disorder or obsessive-compulsive personality disorder. The patient has an insomnia problem but does not meet the duration criterion for insomnia disorder. She can be given the diagnosis of other specified insomnia disorder because the clinician can specify the way in which her disorder differs from one of the DSM-5 insomnia diagnoses. If the clinician lacked specifying information or had reason to choose not to provide specification, the diagnosis would be unspecified insomnia disorder.

Other Specified Insomnia Disorder (p. 420)

27. A 74-year-old woman has a history of daytime sleepiness interfering with her ability to carry out her daily routine. She reports that it has become progressively worse over the past year. Polysomnography reveals sleep apnea without evidence of airway obstruction with two or three apneic episodes per hour. What is the most appropriate diagnosis?

    A. Central sleep apnea.
    B. Other specified sleep-wake disorder (atypical central sleep apnea).
    C. Unspecified sleep-wake disorder.
    D. Rapid eye movement (REM) sleep behavior disorder.
    E. Circadian rhythm sleep-wake disorder.

    Correct Answer: B. Other specified sleep-wake disorder (atypical central sleep apnea).

    Explanation: The patient does not meet full criteria for central sleep apnea because her apneic episodes occur at a frequency of fewer than five per hour. This deviation from diagnostic criteria can be specified. Therefore, "other specified" rather than "unspecified" sleep-wake disorder is the appropriate diagnosis.

    Other Specified Hypersomnolence Disorder (p. 421)